Psychiatry and Philosophy of Science

Philosophy and Science

Series Editor: Alexander Bird

This new series in the philosophy of science offers fresh treatments of core topics in the theory and methodology of scientific knowledge and introductions to new areas of the discipline. The series also seeks to cover topics in current science that raise significant foundational issues both for scientific theory and for philosophy more generally.

Published

Philosophy of Biology
Brian Garvey

Psychiatry and Philosophy of Science
Rachel Cooper

Theories of Scientific Method
Robert Nola and Howard Sankey

Forthcoming titles include

Empiricism
Stathis Psillos

Models and Theories
Roman Frigg

Philosophy of Chemistry
Robin Hendry

Philosophy of Physics
James Ladyman

Psychiatry and Philosophy of Science

Rachel Cooper

McGill-Queen's University Press
Montreal & Kingston • Ithaca

ISBN: 978-0-7735-3386-8 (bound)
ISBN: 978-0-7735-3387-5 (pbk.)

Legal deposit fourth quarter 2007
Bibliothèque nationale du Québec

Published simultaneously in the United Kingdom by Acumen Publishing Limited
and in North America by McGill-Queen's University Press

Library and Archives Canada Cataloguing in Publication

Cooper, Rachel Valerie
Psychiatry and philosophy of science / Rachel Cooper.

(Philosophy and science)
Includes bibliographical references and index.
ISBN 978-0-7735-3386-8 (bound)
ISBN 978-0-7735-3387-5 (pbk.)

1. Psychiatry--Philosophy. 2. Science--Philosophy. I. Title.
II. Series: Philosophy and science (Montréal, Québec)

Q175.N652 2007 616.89001 C2007-905553-2

Designed and typeset by Kate Williams, Swansea.
Printed and bound by Biddles Ltd., King's Lynn.

Contents

Acknowledgements

A great many people have helped me in writing this book. First, I must thank Jennifer Radden and Tim Thornton, who read the manuscript for the publishers, and both offered many valuable comments. Heather Carrick, Nick Clark-Steel, Andrew Divers, Lindelwe Kumalo and Trevor Steele also all read drafts of the entire book and helped me greatly. Tonia Morton offered helpful advice regarding Chapter 9.

I am also very grateful to my colleagues in the Philosophy Department at Lancaster University (David Archard, Sam Clark, Sean Crawford, Brian Garvey, Neil Manson, John O'Neill, Alison Stone, Cain Todd, and Garrath Williams). They have all been generous with both their time and advice. Collectively they read and commented on Chapters 2, 3, 6 and 9, and individually they have also helped me with numerous points throughout the book.

Some parts of this book have previously been published elsewhere as papers and book reviews. Material from Chapter 3 has been published as "Aristotelian Accounts of Disease: What are they good for?", *Philosophical Papers* (2007). Sections from Chapter 4 have appeared as "What is Wrong with the DSM?", *History of Psychiatry* **15** (2004), 5–25. Parts of Chapters 2 and 4 are taken from book reviews on Ian Hacking's *Mad Travelers* and on Richard Freiherr von Krafft-Ebing's *Psychopathia Sexualis* published by the web-based review site *Metapsychology.*

Sections of this book have been presented at conferences as follows: "How do Case Histories Explain?", British Society for the Philosophy of Science conference, University of Southampton (July 2006); "Values and Truth in Psychiatry", International Conference for Philosophy of Psychiatry, Leiden (June 2006); "Disorder, Deviance and Normality – Can Science Distinguish Them?", Royal Institute of Philosophy conference on Philosophy, Psychiatry and Psychology, University of Birmingham (May 2006); "Understanding the Other: Psychiatry as a Test Case", Kuhn and the Sociology of Scientific Knowledge conference, University of Cambridge (March 2006); "What is Wrong with Aristotelian Accounts of Disease?", The Concept of Disease conference, University of Leeds (June 2005). Parts of the book have also been presented at departmental philosophy seminars at the universities of Bristol, Cambridge and Lancaster, and the Open University. I am very grateful for comments made by the audiences at all these events. Lastly, I should like to thank Kate Williams, who copy-edited this book.

1. Introduction: psychiatry and philosophy of science

This book is about psychiatry and the philosophy of science. It aims to be of interest to philosophers of science and their students, to mental health professionals and also to a broader "lay" audience. I have two main objectives. For readers interested primarily in psychiatry I shall show that psychiatry is similar enough to other sciences for ideas from the philosophy of science to be helpful in solving conceptual problems within psychiatry. For readers interested primarily in the philosophy of science I shall show that psychiatry is different enough from other sciences for an investigation of psychiatry to enable old problems in the philosophy of science to be viewed from a new and fruitful angle.

Some readers of this book will be unfamiliar with key concepts in psychiatry. Others will be new to the philosophy of science. The first part of this introduction explains terms and concepts that may be novel. The second part of this chapter considers whether psychiatry can rightly be considered a science. The final section sketches the topics that will be considered in the remainder of the book.

1.1 An introduction to terms and concepts

Here I explain terms and concepts that may be unfamiliar. Some of this introduction will be frustratingly basic to readers who are already familiar with the subject matter, and they will not miss anything important if they skip the introductory sections.

1.1.1 Psychiatry, psychology, psychoanalysis?

Many people are unsure of the differences between psychiatry, psychology and psychoanalysis. In a nutshell, psychiatrists are medically trained doctors who specialize in treating mental illness. Although they may employ "talking cures", as medics they are also able, and often willing, to prescribe psychoactive medication to their patients.

Psychologists, on the other hand, are not medically trained, and are not able to prescribe drugs. Instead they use psychological techniques to help patients. The therapies they employ depend on talking to patients and seeking to modify their behaviour, rather than on direct biochemical intervention. Thus they may counsel patients individually, or lead group therapy sessions, or offer cognitive behavioural therapy, or family therapy, or some such.

Psychoanalysts are distinctive because they belong to one or other of the various schools of thought that have their origins in the ideas of Sigmund Freud. Psychoanalysis has been the dominant approach to helping the mentally ill in various times and places (for example, in the US in the 1960s). Currently, in the UK, however, psychoanalysts are rare, and in the US they are increasingly marginalized. In some countries psychoanalysis is considered a branch of medicine, and all analysts are medically trained doctors. In other countries there are also lay analysts, that is, people who have been trained in psychoanalysis but are not trained in medicine. In traditional psychoanalysis, the patient will be seen for 50 minutes three, four or five times a week. Analysis will normally take two to four years. As it is so time intensive, psychoanalysis is very expensive.

Even in places where psychoanalysts are rare, it is common to find therapists who have been influenced by psychoanalysis and offer "psychodynamic therapy". In many ways, psychodynamic therapy can be seen as a watered-down version of psychoanalysis. The theoretical framework is similar, but in psychodynamic therapy patients will normally be seen less frequently than those undergoing traditional analysis: maybe once a week. Psychodynamic therapy tends to be more problem-focused; the patient will see the therapist until their presenting problems have been alleviated and then stop.

In addition to psychiatrists, psychologists and psychoanalysts, there are also a large number of practitioners who refer to themselves as "counsellors". In the UK, at present, anyone can call themselves a counsellor, and there is no uniformity in the services that they offer.

1.1.2 What is mental illness?

The nature of mental illness is highly contested. Some theorists go so far as to deny that there is such a thing at all (their claims will be considered in Chapter 2). However, if for the moment we lay such possibilities aside and ask what is commonly understood by mental illness we can say that mental disorders are those disorders that affect the mind. Some produce difficulties with mood (or affect), so depression is characterized by low mood, decreased energy and a lack of interest in life, while those who are manic can be highly energetic and feel on top of the world. Other disorders affect a person's ability to reason, so people with schizophrenia may be afflicted with bizarre thoughts and delusions. Other (more controversial) disorders affect the whole personality. People with antisocial personality disorder, for example, have just that, an antisocial personality.

There are a few mental disorders where the cause is well understood. Huntington's disease, for example, is a degenerative disorder that causes movement problems and personality changes in middle age. It is a genetic disease, produced by a mutation on chromosome 4. As another example, some mental disorders are brought about by poisoning; for example, Korsakoff's syndrome is caused by chronic alcohol abuse. In most cases, though, the causes of mental illness are obscure. Many conditions appear to have multifactorial causes. One's risk of developing schizophrenia, for example, appears to be influenced by genetic factors, but is also increased by drug use, complications in pregnancy and social stressors.

1.1.3 Who are the mentally ill and where are they?

In the popular imagination, mentally ill people are locked up in psychiatric hospitals. However, in recent years, in the UK, the US and many other developed countries, most psychiatric hospitals have been closed down. As such, the vast majority of mentally ill people are now treated as outpatients.[1]

In addition to those who have been diagnosed as suffering from a mental illness, there are also large numbers of people who are diagnosable (i.e. if they went to see a psychiatrist they would be given a diagnosis), but who have never had contact with mental health professionals. Some people do not go for treatment because they prefer to self-treat (in the UK, for example, large numbers of people with depressive symptoms self-treat with St John's Wort). Other people avoid mental health services because they do not consider themselves to have a problem. There are people who hear voices, for example, but who do not regard this as problematic and so do not seek medical help (Romme & Escher 1993).

In recent years, "survivor/user/patient" groups have become an increasingly visible presence in debates in the mental health field.[2] Alongside this, deciding to refer to people as "patients", "clients", "users" or "survivors" has become a political choice.[3] In this book I shall use the terms "patient" or "user" in preference to "client" or "survivor". I avoid the term "client" because I think it obscures the social and political context of much mental health care. To call someone a "client" implies that they have some power. In most client–professional relationships the client employs the professional, and the professional acts in their interests. In contrast, in the mental health field, the "client" may be treated involuntarily. Thus some mental health "clients" are only clients in an Orwellian sense. I have also rejected "survivor" – short for "psychiatric system survivor" – as it implies that mental health services do more harm than good, and I do not believe this to be true. "Patient", a term that I shall be using, is also, of course, problematic. For those who know some Greek it carries implications of passivity. Still, there is some evidence that many of those who consult psychiatrists prefer to be called "patients" (McGuire-Snieckus *et al.* 2003). As such, "patient" seems to me one of the least bad options around, and I shall use it here, although I do not intend to imply that "patients" are passive.

1.1.4 What is the philosophy of science?

Philosophy of science is simply philosophy that is directed at questions to do with science. Philosophers of science work on two distinct types of issue. On the one hand there are philosophers who work on problems to do with the nature of science in general; they ask whether theoretical entities exist, whether science seeks the truth, whether there is a scientific method and so on. On the other hand there are philosophers who work on the philosophical problems that arise in each of the individual sciences. So, philosophers of physics worry about possible interpretations of relativity theory and quantum mechanics, and philosophers of biology work on conceptual problems related to defining species and understanding evolutionary theory. Although it is concerned with psychiatry, the topics dealt with in this book straddle this divide. Some are standard topics in general philosophy of science that are discussed with special reference to psychiatry. Others lie squarely within the philosophy of psychiatry proper. Explaining in greater detail how philosophers of science go about their work is difficult, because there is no one type of question that they ask, nor is there any one type of method that they use. As such, rather than explaining what the philosophy of science is like, I shall instead demonstrate what it is like through the course of the rest of the book.

Those who are new to philosophy may find it helpful to note one key respect in which philosophy differs from other disciplines. Philosophy is more a style of thinking than a body of knowledge. This book consists mainly of arguments that will seek to persuade you of various conclusions. As you read it you should think about the arguments for yourself; ask whether the premises seem plausible, and whether the conclusions follow. It is worth noting that if this book had been written by another philosopher they would almost certainly have drawn quite different conclusions. My aim is not to convey a body of "philosophical facts about psychiatry" but rather to provide an example of how problems in psychiatry might be thought about from a philosophical point of view and how such an approach might prove useful.

1.2 Is psychiatry a science? And who cares?

1.2.1 Why does it matter whether psychiatry is a science?

Within our culture the sciences are granted special status. Scientific experts are deferred to by policy-makers and private citizens alike. Science is taught in schools, and research in the sciences is funded by government bodies and charities. As a consequence, whether a particular field qualifies as a science is a matter of importance and, as such, is frequently hotly contested. Consider, for example, debates over the status of creationism or "intelligent" design. Proponents argue that these are "scientific" theories, and as such should be taught in schools alongside evolutionary theory. On the other hand, in the words of an article in the *Guardian* newspaper, "Critics argue that intelligent design cannot be classed as science. It cannot be tested, and is therefore merely a philosophical concept" (Seward 2005). Science has a higher status than philosophy and the other humanities, and a far higher status than fields considered to be "pseudo-sciences", such as astrology and homeopathy. Whether psychiatry counts as a science is thus a question of practical importance. If psychiatry is a science then it will be better funded and psychiatrists will be granted greater authority than if it is not. In addition, whether psychiatry can be considered a science matters for my project here: if psychiatry is a science then it is more likely that applying ideas from the philosophy of science to conceptual problems within psychiatry will prove fruitful.

1.2.2 Popper and demarcation

The problem of distinguishing science from pseudo-science (the "demarcation" problem) was most famously discussed by Karl Popper (1963), one of the greatest twentieth-century philosophers of science. Popper will be familiar to many of those interested in the question of the scientific status of psychiatry as he is well known for his attacks on psychoanalysis. In his youth Popper was greatly impressed by the then fashionable theories of Marxism, Freudian psychoanalysis and Adlerian psychology. However, as time passed he became increasingly frustrated with these areas. The problem as he saw it was that Marxism, psychoanalysis and Adlerian psychology accounted too easily for all possible happenings. As illustration, Popper asks us to consider how a Freudian might explain a man's response to a drowning child. Suppose the man risks his life and rescues the child. The Freudians can explain this: the man has achieved sublimation. On the other hand, suppose the man pushes the child under. In this case, Popper says, the Freudians can cope equally well; they will say that the man suffers from repression (*ibid.*: 35). Indeed, Popper claims, we cannot think of any possible human behaviour that cannot be explained using Freud's theories.

In contrast, consider a theory such as Einstein's theory of relativity. There are experimental findings that concur with predictions from Einstein's theory: Einstein predicted that light must be attracted by heavy bodies (such as the sun). As such, the light from stars will be slightly shifted from the line we might expect. Usually this effect cannot be detected because light from the sun makes light from the stars invisible. During a solar eclipse, though, the effect can be measured and, as it happens, it fits with Einstein's theory. For Popper, the noticeable thing about Einstein's prediction is that it is so risky. Einstein predicts a very particular effect, one that no one had previously expected. Rather than being able to explain whatever the experiment finds, Einstein has committed himself: one possible result, and one possible result only, can be accommodated by his theory.

Thinking about Einstein's and Freud's predictions led Popper to propose his famous criterion of falsifiability for distinguishing science from pseudo-science. According to Popper, a scientific theory is one that is falsifiable: in other words it is possible for it to be proved false. A scientific theory cannot explain all possible happenings, but takes risks. Having made a risky prediction, the observations may fit with the theory, in which case, for the time being, it can be maintained. On the other hand, the world may not turn out to be as the theory predicts, in which case the theory must be abandoned and a new theory constructed. In contrast, a pseudo-scientific theory is not falsifiable: whatever happens, the theory will be able to account for it.

As previously noted, Popper counted psychoanalysis as a prime example of pseudo-science. Following Popper's work, a minor academic industry has devoted itself to assessing the fairness of Popper's critique of psychoanalysis. In *The Foundation of Psychoanalysis* (1984) Adolf Grünbaum argues at great length that Popper is wrong and that many of the claims of psychoanalysis are in fact falsifiable. As Grünbaum points out, there are passages in his writings where Freud explicitly sets out the kinds of evidence that would falsify his theory. Thus, Freud held that paranoia only occurs as a consequence of repressed homosexual love, and writes that if a case of paranoia emerged in which there were no such repressed desires then he would abandon his theory. In other places, Freud actually abandons a theory in the face of recalcitrant evidence. Grünbaum concludes that Popper's attack on psychoanalysis is unfair. Psychoanalysis may have been falsified (and so be a false scientific theory), but it is not unfalsifiable (so it is at least a scientific theory).[4]

With the passage of time, interest in the question of the falsifiablity of psychoanalysis has decreased. At least in part this is because most philosophers of science now reject Popper's demarcation criterion. One of the major problems for Popper's theory is caused by the Quine–Duhem problem (a similar, if not identical problem, is also known as the experimenter's regress) (Duhem 1954; Quine 1961; Collins & Pinch 1993). The problem is that many factors can affect the outcome of an experiment. For an experiment to give the result predicted by a theory it is not merely the case that the theory must be correct. The equipment involved also has to be working properly, and any statistics have to be interpreted correctly. As such, when an experiment yields a result that goes against the theoretical prediction one cannot simply conclude that the theory is false. It might be that there is a problem elsewhere: maybe a wire has come loose, maybe the calculations are wrong. To complicate things further some of the factors that might interfere with the results might as yet be unknown. As such, when one gets an unexpected result this does not prove that the theory is false; something (possibly as yet unknown) might have gone wrong elsewhere.

To be fair, Popper himself is alert to such difficulties, and amends his account to deal with them. He writes that scientists should agree beforehand how they will interpret results (1959: §20). That is, they agree beforehand that if their experiment gives a result that does not fit their theory they will, say, check the wires and the calculations, but not resort to claiming that unknown factors are interfering with their results. With such amendments much of the intuitive attraction of using falsifiability as a demarcation criterion is lost, however. Whether a theory is scientific depends no longer on matters of pure logic (does it make falsifiable predictions regarding observables?), but on the attitudes of the practitioners (is this or that possible intervening factor worth worrying about?).

Following Popper, various other philosophers have proposed different demarcation criteria. Most famously, Thomas Kuhn (1970) suggested that a field becomes scientific when its practitioners find their first paradigm. We shall discuss paradigms further in Chapter 6. But for now we can say that a paradigm provides a structure for thinking about problems. All those who work within a paradigm will agree on what counts as good research; they agree on the questions to be asked, the methods to be used in answering them, and on what kinds of possible solutions will count as satisfactory. When working within a paradigm, scientists engage in "normal science" – they fiddle around making minor improvements – or "puzzle-solving", but they never question the main structure within which they work. Scientists working within the paradigm of Newtonian mechanics, for example, assume that Newton's laws are right. The fundamental theoretical claims of the paradigm are not questioned. Instead of worrying about basic theoretical questions, scientists working within the paradigm solve puzzles: they might show how the paradigm can be extended to a new area and, for example, work on applying the laws of mechanics to the flow of liquids; or they might refine the equipment needed to measure theoretically important results and aim, for example, to measure *G*, the gravitational constant, with ever greater accuracy.

Kuhn suggests that science can be distinguished from non-science as only within science can one find paradigms and the puzzle-solving activities characteristic of normal science. However, Kuhn's criterion has itself come in for criticism. As Paul Feyerabend (1970) points out, there seem to be many non-scientific fields that share the characteristics of normal science. Feyerabend asks us to consider organized crime. Like the scientist practising normal science, a safebreaker also "keeps foundational research to a minimum" (*ibid.*: 200). Like scientists, once safebreakers have found a method that normally works, they are content to merely refine it to deal with new problems. Intellectual puzzle-solving within a taken-for-granted framework is not solely characteristic of science.

1.2.3 Giving up on demarcation: science as a family resemblance term

Finding a demarcation criterion for science is problematic. But maybe the search is misguided. In common with many other recent writers (Dupré 1993; Pickstone 2000) I shall suggest here that no demarcation criterion can be found because "science" is best regarded as a family resemblance term, in the sense introduced by Ludwig Wittgenstein.

In a famous passage in his *Philosophical Investigations*, Wittgenstein asks us to think about what games have in common (1953: §66). He argues that there is no one feature that all and only games possess. Most games have a winner, but some do not (e.g. catch). Many are played with other people, although some are played alone (patience). Some have rules, some do not (cops and robbers). Some are fun, a few deadly serious (Russian roulette). However, although there is no one feature that all games share, games do resemble each other. They resemble each other much as the members of a family resemble each other. When we look at a family photograph we can often see that members are similar even though there is no one feature they all share: some, but not all, have the family smile; some, but not all, a particular chin; some, but not all, a characteristic stance. Nevertheless the members of the family are recognizable because a network of overlapping similarities unites them. There is no one essential feature that any must possess, but each is similar enough in a variety of ways to the others to be recognizable as a family member. Following Wittgenstein, any term that refers to a group of entities that are united by a network of similarities, but which share no one essential feature, is called a "family resemblance" term.

"Science" can be considered a family resemblance term because there is no one feature that defines a field as being a science. Rather, the different sciences are united by a set of overlapping similarities. So many, but not all, sciences posit theoretical entities; many, but not all, provide law-based explanations; many, but not all, use experiments; and so on.

Characteristically, some of the cases that fall under a family resemblance term will be better examples of the kind than others. Consider games. Some games are good examples of "game", in that they possess all the features associated with games. Monopoly, for example, has a winner, is played with a number of people, is fun and there are rules. Other examples of "games" are more tenuous. Is someone turning cartwheels playing a game? No definite answer can be given. Turning cartwheels has some features characteristic of games – it can be done for fun, by children, to pass the time – but are these enough to make it a game? The answer is unclear.

Similarly, when it comes to science some sciences are prototypical sciences, while the status of other fields is less certain. Thus, physics is a good example of a science: physicists posit unobservable theoretical entities; they use laws to make predictions; they experiment; physics can be applied in various technologies. The status of psychiatry is less certain. Psychiatry has many features in common with some other sciences, most obviously psychology and neurology. With other sciences, such as physics, it shares less, but there are still some common features. Still, the fundamental claim of this book is that psychiatry is enough like more prototypical sciences for it to be useful for a philosopher of science to consider it. The remainder of the book will be devoted to establishing this claim.

1.3 An overview of the themes of the book

In what follows I shall examine in greater detail the ways in which psychiatry is like, and unlike, prototypical sciences. I have picked out four features of psychiatry that distinguish it from many other sciences. Examining these characteristics will be a key task in the remainder of the book.

- *The subject matter of psychiatry is contested.* There are many theorists who claim that mental illness does not exist. In so far as the very domain of psychiatry is contested, psychiatry is unlike most other sciences. Chapters 2 and 3 ask whether mental illness is real.
- *Psychiatry employs particular modes of explanation.* Psychiatry makes frequent use of natural history based explanations (i.e. explanations where the nature of a specific case is explained by saying what kind of case it is), and of explanations that depend on individual case histories. Chapters 4 and 5 examine how these forms of explanation operate.
- *Mental health professionals work within different theoretical frameworks.* Most scientists only ever talk to scientists who share their basic theoretical assumptions. In Kuhnian terms, in most areas of science there is only ever one paradigm in a sub-discipline. In contrast, mental health professionals frequently work in multidisciplinary teams in which people have very different theoretical outlooks. Chapters 6 and 7 examine the problems that this causes. Chapter 6 looks at whether it is possible for those with very

different theoretical outlooks to communicate. Chapter 7 looks at reductionism in psychiatry: how do theories that operate at different levels of explanation relate to one another?

- *Psychiatry is problematically shaped by values and interests.* Psychiatry seems to be more problematically shaped by values and interests that many other sciences. Psychiatrists have a history of diagnosing patterns of behaviour of which they disapprove (homosexuality, female promiscuity, runaway children). Currently, much psychiatric research is funded by big business. Chapter 8 examines the various ways in which psychiatric theory can be value-laden and asks how the problems caused by value-ladenness might be overcome. Chapter 9 looks at the challenges posed by the fact that much psychiatric research aims not only to discover the truth about the world but also to make money for its sponsors.

These will be the themes of the book. Through them we shall see how the philosophy of science can be of use in exploring conceptual issues in psychiatry, and how psychiatry can provide fruitful case studies for the philosophy of science.

2. The nature of mental illness 1
Is mental illness a myth?

Unlike most sciences, the basic subject matter of psychiatry is contested; there are many theorists who have claimed that mental illness does not exist. The "antipsychiatrists" of the 1960s are the best known among those sceptical of the category of mental illness. The antipsychiatrists were a diverse group, united only in their suspicion of psychiatry. Each had different reasons for rejecting the category "mental illness": David Rosenhan (1973) claimed that psychiatrists cannot distinguish the sane from the mentally ill; Thomas Szasz (1960; 1972) claimed that psychiatrists wrongly label social misfits; R. D. Laing and A. Esterson (1970) argued that schizophrenics are fundamentally normal individuals who are made scapegoats by their families; Michel Foucault (1971) argued that "mental illness" is a historically contingent category. Although the antipsychiatrists had different reasons for rejecting the category of mental illness, in every case the basic thought is that judgements of mental illness are radically unstable (varying with perceiver, historical period or social context) and that this throws the reality of mental illness into question. In this chapter I shall examine, and ultimately reject, the antipsychiatrists' arguments.

2.1 Is mental illness in the eye of the psychiatrist?

In 1973 Rosenhan published his famous paper "On Being Sane in Insane Places". Rosenhan had persuaded eight sane people to see whether psychiatrists could distinguish them from the insane. The pseudo-patients told hospital admissions staff that they heard a voice that said "thud". All eight were promptly admitted. Once admitted, the pseudo-patients acted as normally as they could within the hospital environment. Despite this, the subjects were still perceived by hospital staff as mentally ill. Within the context of the mental hospital, their normal behaviour was interpreted as manifesting psychopathological disturbance. For example, a "patient" who kept notes of his experiences was described as indulging in "excessive writing activity". Each pseudo-patient was detained for between seven and fifty-two days. Even on release they retained a diagnosis: "schizophrenia – in remission". It seems that the hospital staff considered the subjects to be mentally ill because that is what they expected.

Many have taken Rosenhan's study to show that psychiatrists are charlatans. They claim to be experts on mental illness, but cannot distinguish the sane from the mad. Others have attempted to defend psychiatry by saying that improved systems of psychiatric diagnosis at least mean that the Rosenhan study could not now be repeated.

Whether Rosenhan's study can be repeated today is currently under dispute. Lauren Slater (2004) may or may not have repeated Rosenhan's experiment, and may or may not have found substantially the same results. Slater (2004) reports that she presented herself at eight different psychiatric emergency rooms and, like Rosenhan's pseudo-patients before her, claimed to have been hearing a voice saying "thud". Slater was not admitted to any hospital. But she says she was given a diagnosis – depression with psychotic features – and prescribed both antipsychotics and antidepressants to treat it. She concludes that psychiatrists can still be persuaded to diagnose the normal. All that has changed is that they now admit fewer patients into hospital and are less fond of the diagnosis of schizophrenia. Since the publication of her book, however, other authors have failed to confirm Slater's findings (Spitzer *et al.* 2005), and Slater has been accused of fraud (Zimmerman 2005). In response, Slater (2005) claims she is under attack from "a gang of psychologists and psychiatrists" who are setting out to discredit her.

Luckily we need not determine the truth here. I shall argue that even *if* Rosenhan's study can be repeated today, it would fail to demonstrate that psychiatrists do not know mental illness when they see it. I shall argue that this conclusion does not follow because those who seek to draw it implicitly rely on a faulty notion of what it takes to know something. Thinking that the Rosenhan study shows that psychiatrists are charlatans implicitly relies on the idea that genuine knowers of a kind must be able to distinguish that kind from *all possible* look-alikes. But, I shall suggest, this is too high a demand. Rather, in order to know that something is of a kind we just need to be able to distinguish that kind from *relevant* look-alikes.

Consider the following story told by the epistemologist Alvin Goldman (1976). Suppose that Henry is driving along with his young son. Together they label the objects that they pass: "There's a cow", "There's a tractor", "There's a barn". In the normal course of events we have no doubt that Henry here displays knowledge. For instance, he knows that there is a barn. We take Henry to be a reliable barn-detector because he can distinguish barns from relevant look-alikes; he knows that the object is not a house, or a windmill, or a church – it is a barn. But now let us change the scenario somewhat. Suppose that Henry and his son enter new territory. Unknown to them they drive into Fake Barn Land, a place where under-employed philosophers have constructed dozens of papier-mâché barn facades. When viewed from the road these look like barns, but they are not barns; they are just barn facades, held up with scaffolding at the back. Henry and his son continue their game: "There's a horse", "There's a windmill", "There's a barn". This time, however, we do not think that Henry knows that he is seeing a barn. There are multiple fake barns around. He could so easily be tricked that his barn beliefs are no longer secure. In Fake Barn Land he is no longer a reliable barn-detector.

The conclusion that Goldman draws is that Henry knows barns when he sees them in normal country, but not when he is in Fake Barn Land. To know something one needs to be able to distinguish it from relevant look-alikes, and in different contexts a different range of possible look-alikes are serious candidates for causing confusion.[1] In normal contexts, to know something one only needs to be able to distinguish it from other things that might realistically cause confusion. So, for me to know one of a pair of identical twins I will need to be able to distinguish her from her pair reliably. The other twin is a serious candidate for misidentification and I need to be able to discount the possibility that I am looking at the wrong one. On the other hand I do not need to be able to distinguish the twin from all logically possible look-alikes. I *might* have been tricked by an evil surgeon who has surgically altered an impostor to look like the twin, but this is not a serious possibility and I do not need to worry about it.

How does this apply to the Rosenhan study? It suggests that we should consider psychiatrists to know mental illness when they see it if they can distinguish the mentally ill from other relevant look-alikes. Between 1973 and 2004, nine out of the many thousands who presented at psychiatric emergency rooms were doing a Rosenhan-style study. Such journalists are as rare as fake barns in normal country. Thus, journalists who are pretending to be insane do not count as relevant look-alikes in normal contexts, as it is not normally a serious possibility that the person being examined by the psychiatrist is just a journalist. Rather, in normal contexts relevant look-alikes of the mentally ill are those kinds of people that a less than competent psychiatrist might regularly confuse with the mentally ill. They would include people with symptoms caused by physical disorders, criminals who are pretending to be insane to avoid going to prison, visitors and trainee psychiatrists. In normal contexts, a psychiatrist who can distinguish mentally ill people from these relevant look-alikes is a reliable detector of mental illness. And, I suggest, over the years psychiatrists have developed techniques for distinguishing these relevant look-alikes from people who are mentally ill.

Thus, I conclude that the Rosenhan study does not show that psychiatrists do not know insanity when they see it (in normal contexts). It shows that psychiatrists can be tricked, but then who cannot? And, it suggests that if you do not want to be locked up you should not claim to hear voices.

2.2 Is mental illness a historically unstable category?

Of the antipsychiatrists, Foucault is the subtlest and most important. His work is open to multiple possible interpretations, and interested readers should try to read one of Foucault's works on psychiatry for themselves. As I read him, Foucault argues that the concept of "mental illness" has a particular history and may never have emerged if our past had been somewhat different. If he is right this undermines the taken-for-granted reality of mental illness.

Foucault's key work on psychiatry comes in both a long and a short version. *Madness and Civilisation* (1971) is the short version, and for a long time it was the only one available in English. As such, much of the secondary literature in English focuses on this version. More recently, the long version has also become available as *History of Madness* (2006).

Foucault's key claim in *Madness and Civilisation* is that contemporary notions of mental illness are rooted in contingent, historical developments. The history that has led to our thinking of mental illness in the way that we do could easily have been different, and if it had been different, our current ways of thinking would never have arisen. Foucault tells us that prior to the Enlightenment the mad were primarily seen as being odd as opposed to ill. Often mad people were tolerated, and on occasion they were considered gifted. With the Enlightenment, however, being "reasonable" took on a new importance. Society was no longer prepared to put up with "unreasonable" people who did not work, and so all such people were shut away in huge institutions. Most of this mixed group of the delinquent and difficult could be put to useful employment, but the mad could not. As the mad thus formed a residual problem population, they became visible as a group for the first time. Various professions then fought for control over madness. Eventually, the medical profession won in these struggles, and "the mad" came to be reconceptualized as "the mentally ill" as we know them today.

In *History of Madness*, Foucault's account is more nuanced. In this version it is made clearer that seeing madness as a medical problem is not an entirely post-Enlightenment phenomenon. Rather, there have always been strands of thought that have thought of madness as illness. Still, the fundamental message remains the same: according to Foucault there are possible ways of thinking whereby madness does not appear equivalent to mental illness, that is, where madness does not seem like a kind of illness best treated by doctors.

If Foucault is right, then the fact that we think of the "mentally ill" as constituting a medical kind is due to contingent historical factors. If history had worked out differently, a different professional group might have retained or gained control of madness, and we would have ended up thinking about the mad quite differently. Conceivably, for example, the clergy might have won control of madness. Then it is likely that we would have ended up thinking of madness as a mishmash of personal, social and spiritual problems.

Many have criticized Foucault on the grounds that his history is slapdash (e.g. Reznek 1991: 126–7). Some of this criticism is misdirected. Until recently only *Madness and Civilisation* was available in English, and the version now available as *History of Madness* is more textured.[2] In any event, criticizing Foucault on matters of detail misses the philosophical point of his work. If Foucault is wrong about the places, times and people who have thought differently about madness this does not much matter. So long as his history is good enough to establish that it is possible to think of madness in non-medical terms (i.e. by showing that some people somewhere have successfully done so) his philosophical point that our own conceptualization is contingent will be made.

In assessing Foucault's claims it is important to note that he does not think that only our concept of mental illness has a particular history. Although it does not come out very clearly in his work on psychiatry, in his other works – especially *The Order of Things* (1970) – it becomes clear that Foucault thinks that all our concepts have histories. In other words, different people at different times have thought quite differently not only about madness but about everything else as well.

For philosophers brought up in the analytic tradition, the Foucault of *Madness and Civilisation*, *The Birth of the Clinic* and *The Order Things* is perhaps best thought of as "W. V. Quine plus history" (philosophers brought up in the continental tradition will dismiss this as a crass oversimplification, but I find it helpful). Quine (1960) claims that there are different world-theories or, in his terms, conceptual schemes that we could adopt to explain and predict our experiences. We think in terms of a world filled with physical objects; others may think in terms of gods and spirits. Alternative schemes might be equally successful in organizing our experience. Foucault is similar. While Quine talks in terms of conceptual schemes, Foucault talks in terms of *epistemes*, but in both cases the fundamental claim is that different peoples have successfully thought in quite different ways. Some key differences between Quine and Foucault should be noted, however. First, Foucault's project is historical, in that he thinks he has shown that peoples think differently at different points in history. Secondly, Foucault thinks that the rules of reasoning themselves have histories, so that, for example, at different times different conclusions may seem to follow from the same premises, and the questions that it seems reasonable to ask can vary.

Admittedly, in *The Archaeology of Knowledge* (1972) Foucault distances himself somewhat from this reading. Here he emphasizes that an episteme should not be thought of as a monolithic all-encompassing worldview that imposes the same style of reasoning across all domains, but is instead more complicated. In *The Archaeology of Knowledge*, Foucault tells us that epistemes shift and evolve and that basic ways of thinking may differ radically between different domains at a single time. Still, the similarity with Quine that I wish to highlight remains; for both thinkers there are alternative, equally successful, ways of thinking about the world.

As I read them, neither Quine nor Foucault is radically sceptical. For Quine it is not wrong to say that the world is full of material objects: that is one way (but not the only way) of making sense of things. Similarly, Foucault does not claim that it is a mistake to think of madness as mental illness. Rather, his claim is simply that there are other ways of thinking of the phenomena that we think of in this way.

At points Foucault seems to suggest that some earlier conceptualizations of madness might have political and ethical advantages. However, it is important to note that although Foucault thinks that *if* history had been different we might have conceptualized madness differently, it is not an option for us now to radically change our ways of thinking. For Foucault, one does not choose the episteme that structures one's thoughts. Rather, persons born at a particular place and time are bound to think in particular ways. As he puts it, "One cannot speak of anything at any time" (1972: 44, see also 209–11). As such, Foucault cannot urge us to replace our concept of "mental illness" with something else. Thus, although Foucault is an antipsychiatrist in that he holds that from a God's-eye point of view there are different possible ways of thinking about madness, he is not an antipsychiatrist in the sense of thinking that we could replace our current conceptualizations with something better now. As thinkers we are trapped in a particular episteme, and radical revisionism is not open to us. Of course, as history unfolds we might come to think in new ways, and this might be ethically preferable, but nevertheless, for Foucault, we cannot intentionally overhaul our current ways of thinking. We have no choice but to think of madness in broadly medical terms.

2.3 Is mental illness a moral, rather than medical, problem?

In *The Myth of Mental Illness* (1972) Szasz argues that mental illnesses do not exist. Talk of "sick" minds is merely metaphorical, and should be taken no more seriously than talk of "sick" societies or "sick" jokes. Szasz thinks that minds cannot literally be sick because he thinks that literal diseases are caused by physical lesions. Talk of "mental diseases", where these are supposed to be diseases that specifically do not have a physical basis, is therefore strictly speaking incoherent.

According to Szasz, so called "mental diseases" are not literal diseases but should instead be understood as intentional communications. So, for example, the hysterical paralysis of a young woman, who ensures via her paralysis that leaving her family is impossible, might be interpreted as signifying her unwillingness to move away from home. Such problems are not problems at the same sort of "level" as physical illness; calling for a doctor to cure them makes no more sense than calling for a television repairman to "fix" the bad programme on television (1972: 11).

Of course, Szasz accepts that some abnormal behaviours are produced by brain problems, so strokes can cause problems with speech, for example. Szasz thinks that such conditions can properly be treated by physicians, but he thinks that as the problem is located in the brain they should be called brain disorders as opposed to mental disorders.

Szasz promotes his ideas as if they were radical. His slogan that mental illness is a "myth" implies that those who treat mental diseases do not treat genuine diseases. As such, according to Szasz, psychiatrists do not practise genuine medicine. Instead they simply help people with problems in living, or, worse, act as agents of social control. Not surprisingly many psychiatrists have reacted angrily to such claims. However, I think that on the most plausible reading Szasz's claims turn out to be fairly moderate, and we can agree with him on many points.

The first point to note is that Szasz agrees that any so called "mental disorders" that turn out to have a biological basis are real diseases. If schizophrenia is discovered to be caused by a genetic defect, or by a neurological abnormality, then Szasz will accept that schizophrenia is a disorder. Szasz prefers to refer to any biologically caused diseases that have psychological symptoms as brain diseases rather than as mental diseases. Still, there is no point quibbling over terminology, and as there is increasing evidence that a great many of the conditions that psychiatrists treat have some kind of physical basis, this means that Szasz will have to accept that much of the time psychiatrists treat real diseases.

Secondly, note that Szasz is surely right in claiming that some behaviours should not be considered symptoms of illness, but are instead purposeful actions for which individuals should be held responsible. We should not think of political dissidents as being mentally ill. With Szasz we can agree that attempts to put medicine in the place of politics and ethics can be dangerous.

What, though, of Szasz's claim that a condition cannot be a genuine disease unless it has been shown to be caused by a physical lesion? Here we should part company. In contrast to Szasz, I suggest that we decide whether behaviour should be considered symptomatic by using a form of argument known as *inference to the best explanation*. Inferences to the best explanation work in the following way: we have some phenomenon to be explained, and there is a range of possible explanations. We decide which is the best explanation (most probable, best able to explain all the features of the phenomenon and so on), and we infer that the best explanation is the most likely to be true. For example, suppose I get home and find that the window has been smashed and my television has gone. There is a range of explanations:

- I have been burgled;
- I got drunk last night, smashed the window, pawned the television, and then forgot all about it;
- a freak hurricane broke the window and lifted the television into the air and away.

Of these explanations, the best is that I have been burgled, and so we infer that this is what has happened.

When we are faced with puzzling behaviour we will similarly conclude that the best possible explanation is the most likely to be true. Sometimes the best possible explanation will be a person-level explanation. Such explanations make reference to an individual's reasons, motives and so on. When a person-level explanation is most appropriate, the behaviour comes to be understood as a purposeful action. Assessing such behaviours is the role of ethics and politics rather than medicine. The reason why it is wrong to label a political dissident mentally ill is that a person-level explanation in terms of their motives and beliefs explains their behaviour better than does any other explanation.

In other cases, the best explanation will make reference to *sub-personal* systems. Such explanations characteristically make reference to biological or sub-personal psychological mechanisms. So, someone might have a fit because something has gone wrong with a part of their brain, or they might fail to recognize faces because something has gone wrong with their face-recognition system. Szasz talks as if we need to have cast-iron proof that there is a biological cause before being able to infer that the behaviour is probably symptomatic and caused by a disorder. Here, however, he places the standard far too high. It is reasonable to infer that behaviour is probably symptomatic so long as a sub-personal explanation looks like a *better* explanation than does a person-level explanation. All sorts of evidence short of cast-iron proof may make this the case. For example, a pattern of behaviour may be more commonly seen in a particular biological kind of person (five-year-old boys, say, or menopausal women); behaviours may co-occur in ways that do not make sense from a purposeful point of view (so feelings of depression often co-occur with sleep problems); a pattern of behaviour may fail to "fit" with the rest of a person's life history (as in dissociative conditions, where there are memory lapses between semi-independent pockets of behaviour). All such features tend to make a sub-personal explanation more plausible than a personal explanation. In these cases we can posit that the behaviour is symptomatic (as a reasonable, though fallible, working hypothesis).

In making these claims, I need to be careful. All our behaviours must have some sort of sub-personal explanation. When I get a glass of water because I feel thirsty there will also be a sub-personal explanation in terms of my muscles contracting and so on. For it to be reasonable to conclude that a behaviour is symptomatic, it cannot simply be the case that there *is* a sub-personal explanation of the behaviour (this criterion would render all behaviours symptomatic); rather, the sub-personal explanation has to be substantially *better than* the personal explanation.

Furthermore, I accept that sometimes the best explanation for behaviour will be unclear. Personality disorders stand out as being difficult cases in this regard. People with antisocial personality disorder, for example, have a lifelong history of behaviours such as aggression, recklessness, promiscuity and poor planning and inconsistent work records. Do such people suffer from disorders? Or, are they just troublemakers? The answer is unclear.

In his 1960 paper "The Myth of Mental Illness" (which confusingly shares the title of his book), Szasz claims that mental and physical disorders are radically different. Physical disorders lead to the violation of biological norms, for example, someone's blood pressure might be higher than normal, or their white blood cell count lower than normal. Mental disorders, on the other hand, lead to the violation of psychosocial, ethical and legal norms; someone may fail to pay attention for as long as is expected, or they become angry unacceptably easily. I accept that Szsaz is right in saying that the reasons why physical and mental disorders come to our attention are often different.

Nevertheless, the account given here shows why the nature of the norms that are violated is irrelevant when considering whether a condition should be considered a disorder. Here we have distinguished between problems that are best explained in personal terms and those that are best explained in sub-personal terms. The former problems are ethical or political problems; the latter are potentially medical problems. If someone comes to attention because they violate an ethical norm, for example, they drive recklessly, *but* the best explanation for this norm violation is sub-personal – maybe internal voices are distracting them, or narcolepsy causes them to fall asleep – we consider them to suffer from a disorder. What matters is the nature of the explanation for norm violation, not the nature of the norm that is violated.

We can conclude that Szasz is wrong to suggest that "mental disorder" is a myth. Sometimes the best explanation of a behaviour is sub-personal, and when such behaviours are problematic it may often be reasonable for them to be treated by physicians.

2.4 Do the symptoms of mental illness depend too radically on social context?

Various authors have claimed that the communications of mentally ill people make (more) sense once their social context is taken into account. To the extent that this is true it would suggest that, when considered as an individual, a person diagnosed with mental illness has nothing wrong with them. If the same individual was in a different social environment then they would not be picked out as being insane.

Such a view is most clearly argued for by Laing and Esterson in their *Sanity, Madness and the Family* (1970). This book presents material from hours of interviews with the families of eleven women who have been diagnosed as suffering from schizophrenia. Through an analysis of these interviews, Laing and Esterson argue that schizophrenics are fundamentally normal individuals who have been made scapegoats by their families. They claim that the families of "schizophrenics" present them with confused and impossible demands. So, for example, parents may verbally encourage their children to be independent and to move away from home, but then consistently undermine their attempts to do this. No "sane" response to such demands is possible. When the speech of people who have been diagnosed as schizophrenic is seen within the context of their family situation it makes as much sense as one could expect in the circumstances. It is only when the "schizophrenic" is considered out of context that they seem to act and speak in inexplicably bizarre and irrational ways.

Although Laing and Esterson's study has been influential, I have two reasons for thinking that they demonstrate rather less than they claim. The first is that they only manage to make certain schizophrenic symptoms seem appropriate within the family context. The families that Laing and Esterson examine undermine the confidence of the "schizophrenic" member. Laing and Esterson show that hesitancy in speech and uncertainty in action can be expected from anyone in such a situation. In a few cases, they also manage to make certain "delusions" explicable. In the Abbot family, the "schizophrenic", Maya, believes that her parents are passing coded messages to each other via nods and winks. In their interviews with Laing and Esterson, Maya's parents reveal that they are in fact doing this (although they deny this to Maya). Here, once the family context is understood, Maya no longer appears crazy. However, people with schizophrenia typically also have other symptoms beyond a certain hesitancy and the few delusions that Laing and Esterson manage to explain. If someone hears voices, or sees things that are not there, it is entirely unclear how this can be explained by reference to their family situation.

The second reason why I am not entirely convinced by Laing and Esterson's study is that I am not sure that the families they interview are necessarily all that different from "non-schizophrenic" families. The parents that Laing and

Esterson interview often have peculiar beliefs and are frequently nasty and unsupportive. However, we all know parents like that who do not have schizophrenic children. Originally Laing and Esterson had planned to produce a comparison set of case studies of non-schizophrenic families, but this project was never completed. Thus, as it stands they have offered us eleven cases describing "dysfunctional" families. However, if there are also other families who are just as dysfunctional but that contain no schizophrenic member this matters for Laing and Esterson's claims. Laing and Esterson hold that retreating into the symptoms of schizophrenia is the only option available to the family scapegoat. If scapegoats in other families respond to similar situations in different ways (e.g. by leaving home, or by standing up to their parents) then this weakens Laing and Esterson's argument.

Having said all this I do think that Laing and Esterson are partly right and that it is true that the perceived competence of mentally ill people varies with social context. I shall argue that social forces can operate so as to undermine the conversational competences of the less powerful and marginalized, including mentally ill people, and that this happens quite generally and via a number of mechanisms. First, and most obviously, those with power tend to control the topic of conversation; they then seem more competent because they have the advantage of talking about things they know about and are interested in. Secondly, those with power tend to dominate conversations, this gives them more opportunity to display their competences. Thirdly, those with power are presumed to be more competent, and thus listeners make greater effort to make sense of their puzzling utterances.

As an example, consider how these mechanisms act to make lecturers appear more competent than students. When I teach formal logic I appear to be much better at logic than my students. In part, this is because I *am* better at logic than the average student. Still, my appearance of competence is in large part constructed by the power structures in play. As the lecturer, I get to set all the questions. This guarantees that I can see the point of them. As I selectively set problems that I think I can solve, it also guarantees than I am more likely to be able to solve the questions than my students. Furthermore, I dominate the lecture, and am publicly seen to solve many more problems than my students. Finally, because I am assumed to be competent, when I write something puzzling my audience tries to work out what I intended rather than assuming I have simply made a mistake (so when a symbol of mine is wrong it is a "typo" but when a student's symbol is wrong I mark them down).

As a related example, a number of studies have traced the ways in which the perceived competence of physicians is maintained via communication strategies adopted by members of subordinate groups. Jeremy Greene (2004) looks at the communication tactics employed by pharmaceutical salesmen in post-war America. The problem faced by the "detail men" was that although they knew more about drug use than the physicians they visited they had to pretend to know less; the perceived competence of the doctor as a highly trained professional had to be maintained at all times. The detail men got round this problem by conveying information in convoluted ways. Their training manuals advised them to use phrases such as "I presume you are familiar with X" and "You are aware, I know, that Y, but I should like to take a moment to emphasize Z". Such formulations made it easy for the physician to maintain an appearance of expertise.

Turning to more recent times, Lesley Mackay (1993) has studied contemporary patterns of communication between doctors and nurses. She describes what she calls the "doctor–nurse" game. The problem is that the doctor wants information from the nurse, but in order to preserve status is not prepared to ask for it. Correspondingly, the nurse cannot simply advise the doctor what to do; a nurse who did so would appear uppity. Like the detail men, the nurse has to find roundabout ways of conveying information to the doctor. As Mackay characterizes the game:

> The nurse's knowledge is wanted, but the nurse is not asked for it. Her competence is never revealed, and her opinion is not directly sought. She gains little from the game … The doctor gains in three ways: he receives the coded information, he maintains his own dominant position, and the superior knowledge of nurses can be disguised and overlooked. The rules of this game ensure that the nurse will never win: all the prizes go to the doctor. (*Ibid*.: 173)

The power structures in play ensure that patterns of communication are adopted that shore up the competences of the powerful. Conversely, the competences of the powerless are undermined. In *The Social Construction of Intellectual Disability* (2004), Mark Rapley analyses the conversations that occur between people with intellectual disabilities and those who study them and care for them. Rapley finds that when carers speak to residents in group homes their speech has much in common with that normally directed at animals and babies. The carers dominate the conversation, they adopt simplified language and use a "sing-song" intonation. In addition, Rapley finds:

> an overwhelming reliance by staff upon a set of devices which have a very limited class of preferred seconds [i.e. reasonable replies] – most commonly agreements – which, in and of themselves, cannot but produce the "intellectually disabled" interlocutor as closer to a puppy or a babe-in-arms, than a competent adult conversant. (*Ibid*.: 143)

For example, a carer who wants a resident to set the table says, "Would you like to set the table now since Jim has prepared dinner" (*ibid*.: 167). Here the resident has little option but to agree to the request. Another carer, who is trying to persuade an uncooperative resident to switch medications says, "So you would rather have seizures" (*ibid.*: 150); again, the range of appropriate responses is severely restricted. Faced with such comments the resident has only two choices: they can cooperate with the carer, but note that this gives them no opportunity to exhibit evidence of intelligence; or they can resist the carer, and appear irrational.

In Rapley's study we also see how a *Davidsonian principle of charity* is applied in interpreting the speech of carers but not in interpreting the speech of those who have been diagnosed as suffering from an intellectual disability. According to the philosopher Donald Davidson (1973/4) when we seek to interpret other people we normally apply the principle of charity, that is, when they say something odd, we try hard to make good sense of what they say. This is how we usually manage to make sense of metaphor, sarcasm and so on. Consider this exchange between the mother of an intellectually disabled woman and a researcher:

> Researcher: What do you think it means to have a mental handicap?
> Mother: Hard work. Hard work, frustration and tears.
> (Rapley 2004: 118)

We know that "mental handicap" does not literally mean "hard work". In making sense of the mother's speech we apply the principle of charity. We assume that the mother is knowledgeable and rational and then make the best sense of her claim that we can. Here we conclude that she is telling us what it is like to care for an intellectually disabled child.

In contrast consider the following exchange, this time between a researcher and Kathleen, an intellectually disabled woman:

> Researcher: So what does it mean if you have a mental handicap?
> Kathleen: It means you get made fun of. (Rapley 2004: 125)

Although exactly parallel to the response made by the mother, in interpreting this speech the researchers do not employ the principle of charity. As she has been diagnosed as suffering from an intellectual disability it is not taken for granted that Kathleen is rational and knowledgeable. The researchers conclude that Kathleen does not really understand what mental handicap is and that she does not know that she is mentally handicapped.

Similar problems face people who have been diagnosed as suffering from mental illness. Here the classic case is discussed by Laing in *The Divided Self* (1965). Laing considers a 1905 case study by Emil Kraepelin, the great nineteenth-century German psychiatrist who first distinguished manic-depressive and schizophrenic-type illnesses. Kraepelin is presenting a patient with catatonic excitement to a room full of students. Kraepelin tells us:

> The patient sits with his eyes shut, and pays no attention to his surroundings. He does not look up even when spoken to, but he answers beginning in a low voice, and gradually screaming louder and louder. When asked where he is, he says, "You want to know that too? I tell you who is being measured and is measured and shall be measured. I know all that, and could tell you, but I do not want to." When asked his name, he screams, "What is your name? What does he shut? He shuts his eyes. What does he hear? He does not understand; he understands not. How? Who? Where? When? What does he mean? ..."
>
> (quoted in Laing 1965: 29)

Kraepelin takes the patient's utterances to be symptomatic. In Kraepelin's view the patient has "not given us a single piece of useful information". His talk was "only a series of disconnected sentences having no relation whatever to the general situation" (quoted in *ibid.*: 30). Laing thinks otherwise. He applies the principle of charity and takes the patient to be protesting against being questioned in front of an audience of students. To Laing's ears the patient is "objecting to being measured and tested. He wants to be heard" (*ibid.*: 31). Whether one applies the principle of charity produces a gestalt shift in the way in which we perceive the speech. As Laing puts it, "this patient's behaviour can be seen in at least two ways, analogous to the ways of seeing vase or face" (*ibid.*).

The point of all this is that people's perceived competence depends to a large extent on the conversational strategies adopted by those who talk to them. These strategies tend to favour the powerful and undermine the powerless. Thus, the conventions that govern conversation ensure that if one is a physician or a lecturer it is frequently hard to go wrong, but conversely, if one has been diagnosed as intellectually disabled or mentally ill, it is often hard to appear competent. Having said all this, I do not think it is sufficient to show that mental illness and intellectual disability do not exist. I suggest that a person's perceived competence is amplified or undermined, but not entirely created, by the conventions that govern conversation.

2.5 Can mental illness be viewed as a good thing?

After his work with Esterson, Laing went on to develop a different account of schizophrenia. In *The Politics of Experience and the Bird of Paradise* (1967) he claims that schizophrenia should not be considered pathological because it is a good thing. According to Laing, people with schizophrenia are potentially better off than "normal" people. Normal people have constructed a false self to present to the world. From early childhood, normal people are trained to act in a way that does not reflect their true experience of life. So, for example, children are made to pretend to be grateful for presents that they do not like. Later, they are forced to be polite to teachers and employers, no matter how unreasonable and unfair their demands. Under such pressures, normal people create a false-self and become alienated from their own experiences.

People who refuse to construct a false-self are called "schizophrenic" by the rest of the population. However, according to Laing, "schizophrenic" people are less alienated from themselves and potentially better off than everyone else. Schizophrenic experiences are part of a healing spiritual journey that can potentially lead schizophrenic people away from normality and into a higher form of sanity.

Unfortunately, Laing continues, modern psychiatric treatment tends to interfere with the mystical journey of schizophrenics. When schizophrenics are "treated" instead of being allowed to progress through their journey, they can become stuck in a limbo-like state, neither "normal" nor "truly-sane" but merely messed up and confused. Laing thinks that ideally psychiatric hospitals should be replaced with retreats in which schizophrenics can be permitted to journey through psychosis in safety, perhaps with the help of a guide to "inner space", an ex-patient who has successfully navigated the voyage themselves.

Laing summarizes his view (in typical Laingian-style) thus:

> The madness that we encounter in "patients" is a gross travesty, a mockery, a grotesque caricature of what the natural healing of that estranged integration we call sanity might be. True sanity entails in one way or another the dissolution of the normal ego, that false self competently adjusted to our alienated social reality: the emergence of the "inner" archetypal mediators of divine power, and through this death a rebirth, and the eventual re-establishment of a new kind of ego-functioning, the ego now being the servant of the divine, no longer its betrayer. (1967: 119)

The Politics of Experience has been hugely influential, but I find it hard to fully understand why. The book is written in a rambling style, and makes constant reference to mystical thinking. Nothing I can say will dissuade Laing's supporters of the value of his views. The best I can do is to point out the metaphysical extravagance of Laing's account of schizophrenia. Anyone who wants to adopt Laing's account is committed to many claims that on the face of it appear implausible. The Laingian has to believe that there is some kind of mystical world beyond the everyday, and that psychotic experiences enable one to get in touch with it. There is simply no good reason to believe this. Less extravagantly, one might conclude that things are roughly as they appear, that is, there is one world (the everyday world) and many of those diagnosed with schizophrenia have problems navigating it.

All this being said, and while I see no reason whatsoever to think that schizophrenia is a mystical journey to a higher form of sanity, I do think that occasionally schizophrenia can be a good thing. Some people diagnosed with schizophrenia like having hallucinations and hearing voices. One person says this about his hallucinations:

> Hallucinations can be good or bad. The world can be transformed into heaven or hell at the drop of a hat … The plus side to them is certain moments of vividness that can turn a walk through a park, or whatever, into a walk through paradise … (Romme & Escher 1993: 130)

> It's a type of drug, something that people would pay money for … I consider myself the luckiest of individuals, and am most pleased with this mind … My life is an adventure, not necessarily safe or comfortable, but at least an adventure. (*Ibid.*: 133–4)

As another example, a friend of mine with schizophrenia told me that he heard voices that told him funny jokes. Now, of course, that someone says that they like being the way they are is not sufficient to show that they have a good life. Someone who believes he is God's prophet may think he has a good life (he has been chosen for a special mission and so on), but if we think he is deluded we will consider him pitiful. He is pitiable because he believes himself to be engaged in valuable projects that are not actually valuable. Still, if someone sees bright colours in a park, or hears funny jokes, there does not seem to be any such potential problem. Seeing beautiful things and hearing funny jokes are uncomplicated benefits.

Here we must be careful, as in addition to having odd sensory experiences many people with chronic schizophrenia suffer from cognitive deficits (Lewis 2004). If those with pleasant hallucinations also suffer cognitive deficits then their condition might be a bad thing overall. Still, not all people with schizophrenia suffer cognitive problems. As such, there may be some people for whom schizophrenia has no bad effects.

Thus possibly schizophrenia can sometimes be a good thing. Where I part company with Laing is that he thinks that it is always a good thing to have schizophrenia, while I think that schizophrenia will only rarely be beneficial. In addition, it is worth noting that although schizophrenia may have some positive aspects, most other mental disorders do not. There is simply nothing good about depression, or panic attacks, or anxiety, for example.

2.6 Conclusion

In this chapter I have looked at the arguments of the antipsychiatrists and argued that they are insufficient to throw doubt on the existence of mental disorder. At this point it may be useful to briefly summarize the arguments.

We started with Rosenhan's study and saw that this does not show that psychiatrists do not know mental illness when they see it. Those who seek to draw such a conclusion go wrong because they implicitly assume that genuine knowers of a kind must be able to distinguish that kind from all possible look-alikes. But, this is too high a demand. Rather, in order to know that something is of a kind we just need to be able to distinguish that kind from relevant look-alikes. In normal contexts, psychiatrists can be said to know mental illness if they can distinguish the mentally ill from look-alikes such as people with physical conditions, student nurses and so on, and they can do this.

Foucault claims that our conception of mental illness is historically contingent. However, even if he is right in claiming that people long ago thought of madness other than as mental illness, on his account such ways of thinking are not currently available to us (as we are constrained to think in accord with the current episteme). Thus Foucault cannot argue that we should change our ways of thinking.

Szasz claims that mental illness is a myth, but he is wrong about this. In cases where the best explanation of a problematic behaviour is sub-personal it is reasonable to consider the behaviour symptomatic. Nonetheless, Szasz is correct in claiming that behaviours that are best explained at the person-level should not be considered indicative of illness.

Laing and Esterson claim that people diagnosed with schizophrenia are merely normal individuals who have been made scapegoats by their families. Their more radical claims cannot be substantiated. However, it plausibly is the case that a person's perceived competence depends to a large extent on the conversational strategies adopted by those who talk to them. These strategies tend to favour the powerful and undermine the powerless, and in particular they tend to undermine the perceived competences of people who have been diagnosed as suffering from mental illnesses. Nonetheless, this point is not sufficient to show that mental illness is unreal.

Laing's suggestion that schizophrenia is a mystical journey to a higher form of insanity is implausible. In a few cases, conditions that are normally considered mental disorders may improve the lives of those with them. Still, many mental illnesses are bad things to have.

Having dealt with the arguments of the antipsychiatrists, in Chapter 3 we go on to consider the nature of mental disorder. If mental illness is not a myth, what is it?

3. The nature of mental illness 2
If mental disorders exist, what are they?

This chapter examines in greater detail the nature of mental disorder. I address two questions: what is the distinction between mental and physical disorders, and what makes something a disorder at all, as opposed to a normal variation or a moral failing, for example?

3.1 The distinction between physical and mental disorders

The first question we must consider is whether mental and bodily disorders should be considered together, or whether they are radically different kinds of condition. As we have seen, some theorists, such as Szsaz, hold that mental and physical disorders are radically distinct (on Szsaz's account, physical disorders are caused by lesions, whereas mental disorders are mere myths). Still, most contemporary accounts of disorder seek to accommodate both mental and bodily disorders together. In this section I shall argue that this is the most reasonable approach to take.

Attempts to draw a clear-cut distinction between physical and mental disorders fall into difficulties. Splitting disorders on the basis of whether they have physical or psychological causes will not work, as many disorders are affected by both psychological and physical causal factors: one's risk of developing schizophrenia is increased by social stressors, and also by drug abuse, birth complications and genetic factors. Many disorders that are generally considered to have physical causes are made worse by stress, for example, allergies and high blood pressure.

Dividing disorders into those that have physical symptoms and those that have mental symptoms will not do either, as many disorders have both psychological and physical effects. So, flu not only makes our noses run, but it also makes us tired and irritable. As another example, people with Down's syndrome have a distinctive appearance and often have heart problems in addition to suffering from learning disabilities.

No plausible way of cleanly distinguishing mental and physical disorders has been proposed. Moreover, when one considers lists of disorders that are generally classed as "mental" and disorders that tend to be classed as "physical" one can see that the distinction between the two is often somewhat arbitrary. Dominic Murphy (2006: 55–6) cites the case of blindness as an example. Vision is usually considered a mental process. Vision is investigated by psychologists, and philosophers of mind take visual sensations to be paradigm cases of mental processes. Still, problems with visual processing are not treated by psychiatrists and are not considered to be mental disorders. Lawrie Reznek (1991: 174) suggests that visual problems are not considered mental disorders because mental disorders have to affect *higher* mental processes (thinking and feeling). But, this will not do, as psychiatrists treat some disorders related to sleep and sexual function, and these disorders affect lower mental processes. Blindness thus remains an odd case. Another peculiarity is that neurosyphilis is now considered a neurological disorder, while Huntington's disease is still taken to be mental, although both have known physical causes (Murphy 2006: 70). Clearly whether a disorder is classed as physical or mental can depend on purely contingent, historical factors.

No plausible way of cleanly distinguishing mental and physical disorders has been proposed, and there is considerable overlap between mental and physical disorders. Consequently, an account of disorder that can accommodate both mental and physical disorders is to be preferred.

3.1.1 A note on terminology

So far I have been talking about "disorders", but now that we are considering physical disorders alongside mental disorders, some clarification about terminology might be useful. Particularly when it comes to physical conditions, in everyday language we often distinguish between diseases, disabilities, injuries, wounds and so on. In certain contexts the differences between these various kinds of medical problem are important. But often they are not. Any of the above can function as an excuse or justify various benefits, for example. As such, we also have an umbrella concept that lumps all these medical problems in together. In this chapter, as in most philosophical work in this area, "disease", "disorder" or "pathological condition" will be used interchangeably as terms for this umbrella concept. Some people find this odd, and would find it more natural to distinguish between diseases in a narrow sense, injuries, wounds, disabilities and so on (categories that are all lumped together under "disease" here).

While I have some sympathy with those who find it strange to describe a broken arm as a disease, using "disease" to encompass all pathological conditions has become so widespread in the philosophical, and indeed medical, discussions of the nature of the pathological, that it is too late to stem the tide at this point. "Disease" will thus be used in a broad sense here.

My aim in the remainder of the chapter is to provide a brief overview of current debates regarding the concept of disease. A great many different accounts have been proposed. Here I shall not examine them all, but shall focus on five accounts. The first three are accounts that I think are wrong. They are all very different and so when considered together give some idea of the range of accounts currently available. The fourth account I shall consider is one that is along the right lines, and the fifth is a look-alike that must be distinguished from it.

3.2 Biological accounts of disorder

Christopher Boorse (1975, 1976, 1977, 1997) is the best known proponent of a purely biological account of disease. Boorse seeks to provide an account whereby whether a condition is a disease depends solely on value-free biological facts. Boorse's starting-point is that we should think of the human body and mind as being composed of numerous "sub-systems". "Sub-system" is to be taken in the broadest sense imaginable. Organs, systems such as the nervous system, and mental modules (if there are any) will all count as Boorsean sub-systems. Each sub-system of the body and mind has a natural function. So, for example, the function of the heart is to pump blood, and the function of our ears is to enable us to hear. When we are healthy all our sub-systems function as they should.

Sometimes, though, a sub-system dysfunctions. Maybe our hearts stops pumping blood. Or maybe our ears no longer enable us to hear as well as we used to. When a sub-system dysfunctions we have a disorder. The account can also be applied to mental disorders. The function of the theory of mind module (if there is such a thing) is to enable social interaction. A dysfunction here might produce the disorder of autism.

Intuitively, Boorse's idea that the parts of organisms have functions, and that diseases are dysfunctions, is easy enough to grasp. However, when one seeks to give a precise account of "function" things get complicated. As some readers will be aware, in the philosophy of biology there is a vast literature on functions, and various different accounts of "natural function" have been proposed. Of the best known positions, those who adopt Cummins-type views (Cummins 1975) claim that the function of a sub-system is whatever it normally currently does that contributes towards the goals of a larger system. On such an account the function of the heart is to pump blood around the body, as this is what hearts currently normally do that contributes to the organism surviving and reproducing. On the other hand, those who favour Wright-style approaches (Wright 1973) think that the function of a sub-system is fixed by its history. In the biological domain, the Wright-function of a sub-system is whatever it was naturally selected to do. On such an account the function of the heart is still to pump blood around the body, but now this is said to be because this is why natural selection has fitted us with hearts.

In many cases, as with the heart example, whether one adopts a Cummins-style approach or a Wright-style approach to functions will make no difference. Sometimes, however, the Cummins-function of a sub-system and the Wright-function of a sub-system can come apart. This happens if a sub-system was selected because it met one need, but is currently used for something else. Some theorists have suggested that flies' wings were originally used as heat-regulating organs and only later came to be used for flying, for example. If we consider the first fly that started to use its wings for flying, the Wright-function of the wings would be heat regulation, as this is what the wings had been selected for, while the Cummins-function would be flying, as this is how the wings contribute to the fly's goals. (In later generations things get more complicated as selective pressures will begin to select for flying wings).

In other work (Cooper 2002) I have argued that there are deep problems with finding an account of normal function that can be used as the basis of a disorder-as-dysfunction account of contemporary human disorders, but we shall not discuss these problems here. The arguments about function get complicated and we can make do without them. For the record, though, Boorse himself favours Cummins-style functions. He thinks the function of a sub-system is whatever it normally currently does that contributes to the organism surviving and reproducing. Others who agree with Boorse that a disorder is a biological dysfunction (e.g. Wakefield 1992a, 1992b, 1999) have favoured Wright-functions, and claim that the natural function of a sub-system is whatever it was selected to do. Here, we need not worry ourselves further about the various accounts of function, as I shall argue that on any of the currently proposed accounts of function all biologically based accounts of the pathological are inadequate. I shall argue, first, that biological dysfunction is not sufficient for disorder, that is, there are some biological dysfunctions that are not disorders. Then, secondly, I shall argue that biological dysfunction is not necessary for disorder either; there are plausibly some disorders where there is no biological dysfunction.

3.2.1 First problem for biological accounts: dysfunction is not sufficient for disorder

I shall argue that dysfunction is not sufficient for disorder using two examples. The first example concerns bee sex. When bees have sex the male bee explodes, and his rear end remains in the female. This results in the death of the male bee. When this happens, from a biological point of view nothing has gone wrong. This is how bees are supposed to work. Presumably, the fact that the rear end of the male gets stuck in the female increases the chances of fertilization, or some such (as hypothesized by Winston 1987). However, despite the fact that when the male bee explodes everything is going to plan, one can doubt that exploding is in the best interests of the individual bee. Imagine that one day a mutant bee is born. This male bee can have sex without exploding. Would we say that such a bee suffers from a disease? The answer is unclear. Even if we suppose that the non-exploding bee is somewhat less fertile than the exploders, the mutation seems to be in the individual bee's best interests.

On its own, the bee example proves little, but it should prompt us to suspect that biological dysfunction may be insufficient for disease. Individual well-being and biological functioning can come apart, and maybe the former is of more importance for the concept of disease than the latter.

My second example is more important and I think shows conclusively that biological dysfunction is not sufficient for disorder. The American Psychiatric Association (APA) stopped considering homosexuality to be a disease in 1973, and few people nowadays would think of homosexuality as a disorder.[1] However, on Boorse's account, wherever there is a sub-system of the body or mind that fails to fulfil its biological function there is a disorder. Whether there is a dysfunction in the case of homosexuality is of course disputed (see e.g. Ruse 1981). Some go so far as to suggest that homosexuality might be biologically advantageous, perhaps for kin-selection type reasons. Still, in the current state of knowledge the possibility that homosexuality is a biological dysfunction cannot be ruled out. Maybe, for example, some sub-system of the mind has the job of ensuring that human beings are sexually attracted to members of the opposite sex, and homosexuality occurs when this system dysfunctions. As there are multiple possible biological models of homosexuality, currently and until there is further evidence, no one can be sure whether or not homosexuality is a dysfunction in biological terms.

Homosexuality may turn out to be a dysfunction. As such, someone who accepts Boorse's account is forced to admit that homosexuality might be a disorder. Boorse himself accepts this; indeed, he thinks that homosexuality is a disorder, although he adds that on his value-free account of disorder this should not be taken to imply that he thinks it is bad to be gay. Many of us, however, would not be happy to take Boorse's line on this. Many of us would want to say that whether or not homosexuality confers some selective advantage is not really the issue. Plausibly, whether or not homosexuality is a disorder does not depend merely on whether there is some biological dysfunction but on whether it is also *harmful*. In contrast to Boorse's claims, those who think that homosexuality is not a bad thing will generally refuse to consider it a disorder regardless of what biological story turns out to be correct. I conclude that the case of homosexuality thus shows that even if a condition is a biological dysfunction this is not sufficient for it to be a disorder.

3.2.2 Second problem for biological accounts: dysfunction is not necessary for disorder

Could we adapt a disorder-as-dysfunction account, such as Boorse's, and claim that a condition is only a disorder if it is a *harmful* dysfunction? This approach to the pathological has been proposed in a number of papers by Jerome Wakefield (1992a, 1992b, 1999). Importantly for psychiatry, it is also the approach adopted in the APA's *Diagnostic and Statistical Manual of Mental Disorders* (DSM), which says that for a condition to be a disorder there must be both a behavioural or psychological syndrome (that is assumed to be caused by a dysfunction) *and* it must be the case that this syndrome generally causes distress or impairment (i.e. it has to be a bad thing) (APA 1994: xxi). Such an account can deal with the case of homosexuality, which caused problems for accounts that claim that a biological dysfunction is necessary and sufficient for disorder. On an account that says that disorders are harmful dysfunctions, in so far as homosexuality is not harmful, it is not a disorder.

However, such an account of disorder cannot be accepted either, as it is not even necessary that a condition be a biological dysfunction for it to be a disorder. This is because in some cases the genetic bases of disorders may confer a biological advantage and thus be selected. In such a situation, from a biological point of view, there is maybe no dysfunction when cases of the disorder occur. This may well be the case with several types of mental disorder. Conditions including manic-depression, sociopathy, obsessive-compulsivity, anxiety, drug abuse and some personality disorders seem to have a genetic basis and yet occur at prevalence rates that are too high to be solely the result of mutations. This has led evolutionary psychologists to suggest that the genetic bases of these mental disorders must be adaptive in some way or other.

The genetic basis of pathological conditions may be selected for a number of reasons. Most obviously, a condition may be selected because it enhances sufferers' biological fitness in some present environment. Linda Mealey (1995) suggests that the genes for sociopathy are selected for this reason. Sociopaths tend to be more violent and promiscuous than other males, and in tough environments these traits may be adaptive. Other conditions might be of no benefit at present but have been biologically beneficial in earlier times. Agoraphobia and other anxiety disorders, for example, may be of no benefit now, but could have been adaptive when human beings lived in more hazardous environments (Marks & Nesse 1994; Nesse 1987). Or a condition might be selected through kin-selection processes. As individuals are genetically similar to their kin, an individual can increase the number of copies of their genes by helping their relatives to breed successfully. Thus, through kin selection, a condition that is of no direct benefit to an individual may be selected because it benefits the individual's relatives. The genetic basis of generalized anxiety disorder might be promoted for this reason (Akiskal 1998). Generalized anxiety disorder causes sufferers to worry a lot, about, among other things, the welfare of their families. While worrying may be of no direct benefit to people with generalized anxiety disorder, it might help their relatives to have someone looking out for them.

All these hypotheses are controversial and any particular one may turn out to be false. Still, in some cases evolutionary models of disorder may turn out to be correct. In any event, that it is *conceivable* that some disorders might be biologically adaptive is enough to show that it is not *necessary* for a condition to be a biological dysfunction for it to be a disease. It makes sense to think that some disorders may be evolutionarily beneficial, and this shows that biological dysfunction is not a necessary component of our concept of disorder.

I have now argued that biological dysfunction is neither sufficient nor necessary for disorder. We must thus abandon biologically based approaches to disorder, and move on to consider alternatives.

3.3 Fulford's action-based account

Bill Fulford considers "illness" to be a more central concept than "disease" or "disorder". In *Moral Theory and Medical Practice* (1989) he presents an account of illness according to which someone is ill if they experience a failure of ordinary action.[2] His account is inspired by the thought that being able to control our bodies and minds in the ways required to act as we wish is hugely important to us. As such, when people find they cannot act in the ways that they usually can, for example they find that they cannot lift up an arm, or where their body moves without them acting, for example they have a fit, they tend to go rushing to their doctors. Conditions that cause "action failure" are thus the proper concern of medicine.

Fulford also recognizes that many illnesses are characterized by various unwelcome sensations – pains, dizziness, nausea and so on – rather than by direct "failures of action". Fulford thinks he can accommodate these illnesses in his action-based account. He says that in these cases people find themselves unable to act so as to stop a sensation that they would normally do something about. For example, normally when people are in pain they move away from the cause, but in the case of pain that indicates that they are ill they cannot do this. Similarly, normally when people are dizzy this is because they have been spinning around in circles, and they can stop this by sitting down, but in the case of dizziness caused by illness the dizziness will not stop.

Thus on Fulford's account illnesses are (i) states that directly interfere with normal action, or (ii) states characterized by unpleasant sensations that cannot be stopped by normal actions. Fulford's account takes illness to be a more fundamental concept than disease or disorder. He provides an account of illness and then explains the concept of disease derivatively. "Disease", according to Fulford, is a term that encompasses conditions that are linked to the production of illness in a variety of ways. For example, conditions may be considered diseases because they tend to produce illness, or because they are conditions that are widely considered to be illnesses, or because they are illnesses where the underlying physiology is known. All diseases, however, are linked in some way to illness, and all illness is linked in some way to action failure.

The main challenge for Fulford's account is to show that it really is the case that all diseases are linked to action failure. In some cases, at least, such a link appears doubtful. Consider disfiguring conditions, for example. These can plausibly be diseases but it is unclear how such states are linked to failures in action. If I am disfigured, then this will not directly interfere with my ability to act. Nor is a disfiguring condition characterized by unpleasant sensations that I would normally do something about.

Fulford's attempt to incorporate illnesses that are characterized by unwelcome sensations is also inadequate. While it may be fair to say that we can normally act so as to stop a pain, this cannot be said of many other unwelcome sensations. Many pathological sensations are not experienced by healthy people at all. Thus it makes no sense to say of distortions of the visual field, or of sensations of depersonalization, that they are sensations that we can normally stop, as normally such sensations are not ever experienced. For these reasons I suggest that Fulford's account must be rejected.

3.4 Aristotelian accounts of disorder

Aristotelian accounts of disorder have been proposed by a number of authors, most notably by Philippa Foot in *Natural Goodness* (2001), and by Chris Megone in several influential papers (1998; 2000). An earlier, though sketchy, account can also be found in Von Wright (1963). Although Foot's work is well known she is concerned mainly with other issues and discusses disorder only briefly, so the discussion here will focus on Megone's work.

The Aristotelian starts by considering what it means to say that a biological organism is a good specimen of its kind. In the case of animals, the Aristotelian account claims that for each species there is a characteristic life cycle. So, in the case of the frog, for example, it is characteristic that frog spawn hatches into tadpoles, which develop into frogs, which eventually produce more frog spawn. A good organism has all the biological equipment it needs to live successfully in the ways characteristic of its kind. So a good frog has a sticky tongue so that it can catch flies, and is attractive to frogs of the opposite sex. Having such attributes makes it more likely that the frog will lead a good froggy life. Of course, even the best frog may be unlucky and fail to lead a good life. Maybe, for example, it gets run over by a car. Having the attributes of a good frog is not an absolute guarantee that the frog will have a flourishing life; it just increases the frog's chances of being successful. While a good frog has the body it needs to increase its chances of living a good life, a frog that does not have the right biological equipment is diseased.

In the case of human beings, things become somewhat more complicated because the flourishing human life has more to it than just reproducing. Like other animals, human beings need certain biological equipment if they are to survive and reproduce, but on Megone's account the flourishing human life is also the rational life. In summarizing his account Megone tells us that: "the human function is … the life of the fully rational animal. Illness is any incapacitating failure to realize (actualize) this human function" (2000: 56). Here we must note that Megone intends "rational" in a very broad sense. For him, the rational human being is not merely one who is good at playing chess and doing sums, but the human being that is fitted to lead a flourishing life; the rational human being is not only intelligent, but has the right values, and can act in the right way. With this in mind we can say that, on Megone's view, the healthy human being has a body and mind that facilitate leading a flourishing life. So, for example, given that human beings are naturally sociable beings, and that a flourishing life thus includes being able to play games and laugh at jokes, someone whose mind does not equip them to take part in such activities, say because they cannot read emotions, would suffer from a disorder.

3.4.1 Problem: Aristotelian accounts are over-inclusive

The fundamental problem with the Aristotelian account is that it is over-inclusive. It fails to distinguish conditions that are disorders from other states that reduce a human's chances of flourishing. Megone has paid some attention to the problem of over-inclusivity, and his claim that illnesses are *incapacitating* failures to function enables him to distinguish disorders from *some* other bad states. So, staying in bed all day simply because one cannot be bothered to get up is a bad state but not a disorder for Megone, because one is choosing to do nothing, as opposed to being incapacitated. However, although it can cope with cases like this, there are also various incapacitating bad states that are not disorders, and these demonstrate that the Aristotelian account is inadequate. I shall discuss these in three classes: biological bad states that are not disorders; social and educational bad states; and vices.

Biological bad states that are not disorders

There are various biological bad states that we do not consider to be disorders. These include states such as being unintelligent and being ugly. (Of course, we do consider learning disabilities and various deformities to be disorders, but I am thinking here of less severe cases). Biological bad states, such as being ugly or unintelligent, harm the individual, often to a greater extent than do minor diseases such as athlete's foot or eczema. They can result in an incapacitating failure to realize a flourishing life. Thus, the first way in which the Aristotelian account is over-inclusive is that the Aristotelian has no means for distinguishing biological bad states, such as ugliness and stupidity, from disorders.

Social and educational bad states

There are various social and educational bad states that harm the individual but that are not disorders. Examples include poverty, illiteracy and social alienation. Megone has the resources to distinguish some such bad states from disorders. For Megone there is a disorder when something goes wrong with a *part* of a human, leading to an incapacitating failure that diminishes a person's chances of leading a flourishing life. Some social, educational and economic bad states are located externally to the afflicted individual, and so can be distinguished from disorders on this basis. Thus, if I am too poor to buy a decent coat, the problem resides in my threadbare clothes rather than in something internal to me.

However, some social and educational bad states *can* be located within the afflicted individual. Consider someone who has an incomprehensible accent, or someone who is illiterate, or a woman who has been brought up to believe that men are her natural superiors. These people's problems reside within them (at least to the same extent as do recognized disorders such as dyslexia, or speech disorders). Thus, such bad states cannot be distinguished from disorders on the basis of their location. Neither can they be distinguished from disorders on the basis of the amount of harm that they cause. As we have already noted, some disorders do little harm, whereas educational and social problems can be life destroying; in text-based societies few people are as disabled as the illiterate. Thus, such educational and social bad states provide us with examples of another set of cases that the Aristotelian cannot distinguish from disorders.

Vices

In the Aristotelian tradition, vices, like disorders on Megone's account, are said to be states that reduce one's chances of having a good life. Megone suggests that vices and disorders can be distinguished on the following basis: "The theoretical distinction between laziness, or any moral vice, and mental illness is that the former is within the agent's power (*hekon*, in Aristotle's terminology) while the later is an incapacitating failure (*akon*, in Aristotle's terminology)" (2000: 63). I shall argue that Megone's supposed distinction will not hold water: vices will give us another set of cases that the Aristotelian cannot distinguish from disorders. Megone claims that vices and disorders can be distinguished in so far as one is responsible for one's vices but not for one's disorders, but as I shall show such a stance is difficult for an Aristotelian to maintain. It should be remembered that the Aristotelian stresses the role of habituation in the formation of character. Once one has a bad character it is not the case that one can suddenly decide to be good and expect this to make an immediate difference to one's actions. To illustrate the problems that this poses let us take the case of Pete, who, we shall suppose, has a bad temper, gets irritated with me and hits me. Now, given that Pete has a bad temper and that I am deeply irritating, it may not be true that at the moment when he hit me Pete could have chosen not to hit me. Given his nature, he may have been bound to thump me in the circumstances.

Still, the Aristotelian will say, Pete is responsible for his character. It is within his power to practise being even-tempered, to avoid aggression-provoking situations and so on, until he becomes a better person. If Pete is bad tempered now, it is because of actions that he chose in the past.

But, if the Aristotelian takes this route a dilemma arises, and the Aristotelian will be caught on one horn or the other. On the one hand, we can question the degree to which Pete is responsible for his character. Our characters start to be formed in childhood. Suppose that Pete's father told him that real men always hit back and reinforced his aggressive behaviour. Then maybe Pete's father rather than Pete is responsible for his current character. On the other hand, suppose it is true that our past selves are responsible for our character. So, let us suppose that Pete is violent because he often chose to fight when younger, and this means he is to blame when he hits me now. The problem here is that our past selves are also often responsible for our health in precisely the same kind of way. So, it might be the case that Pete is not only aggressive because he chose to fight when young, but that he also has lung cancer because he chose to smoke in the past. To the extent that he is to blame for being violent, he will be equally to blame for having lung cancer. Thus the Aristotelian cannot distinguish vices from disorders by saying that we are responsible for our vices but not our disorders. To the extent that we are responsible for our vices (i.e. when they result from bad choices we made in the past) we are also often responsible for our disorders.

I conclude that vices offer another example where Megone's account is over-inclusive. He lacks the resources for distinguishing disorders and vices. As the Aristotelian account cannot distinguish disorders from various other types of bad state it must be rejected.

3.5 Messy accounts

Having looked at various accounts of disease that will not work, we can finally look at accounts that are along the right lines. A number of writers have put forward what I shall call "messy" accounts of disease. Such accounts employ a number of conditions that are jointly considered to be necessary and sufficient for a condition to be a disorder. I call these accounts "messy" accounts because in giving a number of criteria that are jointly necessary and sufficient for a condition to be a disease they lack the simplicity of single-criterion accounts.

In an account of disease that I have previously proposed (Cooper 2002), I suggest three criteria that are jointly necessary and sufficient for a condition to be a disease. Here I will not argue for my account, but present it as an example of the kind of account that will be needed to deal with the issues of over-inclusivity that cause problems for the Aristotelian. Like the Aristotelian I hold that for a condition to be a disease it must be a bad thing, but to this I add that a condition is only a disease if the sufferer is unlucky, and if the condition is potentially medically treatable. When I say that the sufferer of a disease must be unlucky I mean that the sufferer could reasonably have expected to be better off. In nearby possible worlds most people like them are in a preferable state. In saying that a condition must be potentially medically treatable to count as a disease I do not mean that a treatment must currently be available. Rather, the condition must just be the sort of thing where it is reasonable to assume that a treatment will be forthcoming at some point and would be appropriate; the condition is at least the kind of thing where it seems worth doing medical research.

As my account places greater restrictions on what counts as a disease it can deal with the cases that tripped up the Aristotelian. Unlike the Aristotelian account, my account can distinguish social and educational problems from diseases. Such states are not appropriate targets for medical treatment. Rather, they are better ameliorated by economic, social or educational means. Vices can be distinguished from diseases similarly. When someone is vicious the appropriate response is to reason with them, or punish them, rather than treat them.

On my account, biological bad states that are not diseases can also be distinguished from diseases because the sufferer is not unlucky in the right kind of way. If I have dyslexia this counts as a disease because I could reasonably have expected not to have dyslexia: in nearby possible worlds most people who are relevantly similar to me are not so afflicted. Now let us consider the case of short stature. Suppose I am three foot tall. This is plausibly a disorder. The vast majority of people in nearby possible worlds are taller. On the other hand, if I am five foot two inches tall, although I am certainly on the short side, there are far fewer possible worlds in which I am taller. I am unlucky to be five foot two inches tall, but not unlucky *enough* for my condition to count as a disorder.

Thus, in contrast to the Aristotelian, my account of disease offers a more adequate account of our concept of disease. The necessary trick is to add more conditions for a state to count as a disease. Of course, here my account has only been briefly presented, and some will not find it fully convincing, but that will not affect the key point I want to make here. What I want to argue for here is not so much the correctness of my particular extra conditions, but rather that some such extra conditions will be needed. Only by adding more conditions to the Aristotelian account is it possible to distinguish diseases from non-diseases.

There are also other multi-criteria accounts of disorder on the philosophical market. If acceptable, these too might get round the problems faced by the Aristotelian. For example, Reznek has argued that a condition is pathological if and only if it is an abnormal bodily/mental condition that requires medical intervention and that harms standard members of the species in standard conditions (Reznek 1987: 163–4). He takes it that we decide what we will count as abnormal. He says that "abnormal" functions as a call to action, stating that we consider dealing with the harmful condition to be a priority (*ibid.*: 94), and he thinks "medical interventions" can be defined enumeratively, via a list of possible pharmacological and surgical interventions (*ibid.*: 163).

Reznek's account differs from my own in that I argue that to be pathological a condition need only be harmful to the individual, not to standard members of the species. In addition, while Reznek claims that "medical treatment" can be defined enumeratively, I claim that it can only be defined sociologically: while a drug dealer and a physician might hand out the same drugs, only the action of the physician counts as "medical treatment". Finally, while Reznek claims that we decide what counts as abnormal, I claim that whether someone is unlucky depends at least in part on matters of fact: I can only be unlucky if I could reasonably have expected to have been better off (i.e. if there are many people like me in nearby possible worlds who do not have the condition that I have).

As I see it, the fundamental difficulty with messy accounts is that their intrinsic complexity means that they will only prove convincing if fleshed out in some detail. (Crudely, the thought is that all things being equal an account that makes use of three criteria is going to need three times the support that a simpler account would require). Reznek's account is briefly outlined in a book that mainly deals with other issues, and my account has so far been developed only in a paper (Cooper 2002). It is impossible to tell whether a "messy" account will be adequate until one is developed sufficiently to be precise.

3.6 Disorder as a Roschian concept

To finish, it is worth considering one final account of disorder, which has some similarities with the messy accounts proposed by Reznek and me. In a much cited recent article Scott Lilienfeld and Lori Marino (1995) claim that all proposed accounts of mental disorder have been wrongheaded, because it is in principle impossible to give a set of necessary and sufficient conditions for something being a "mental disorder". According to Lilienfeld and Marino, "mental disorder" is a "Roschian concept". By "Roschian concept" they mean something very close to a Wittgensteinian family resemblance concept (Rosch 1975; Wittgenstein 1953: §§66, 67). We met family resemblance terms in Chapter 1, but it is probably worth reminding ourselves what they are. In Wittgenstein's famous example, there are no necessary and sufficient conditions for something being a game: most games have rules, but some do not; most games are fun, but some are not; and so on. Instead of having any one feature in common, games are united by a network of similarities, rather like the networks of resemblances that make family members look alike. While there need not be any one feature that all family members possess, any two members will be similar in a variety of ways. Similarly, necessary and sufficient conditions cannot be given for something being a mental disorder, Lilienfeld and Marino claim. Rather, whether a condition counts as a mental disorder depends on its degree of resemblance to prototypical cases, such as schizophrenia and psychotic depression. Conditions that are sufficiently like these central cases get counted as disorders, but there are no general rules that determine what it takes for something to be a disorder.

Lilienfeld and Marino's paper has been influential. However, their central argument for the claim that "mental disorder" is a Roschian concept is flawed. Lilienfeld and Marino claim that no account of disorder in terms of necessary and sufficient conditions is possible because whether a condition is a mental disorder may be vague: normal anxiety shades into anxiety disorder, normal drinking shades into alcoholism and so on. Typically, whether something falls under a Roschian concept may also be vague, and so Lilienfeld and Marino conclude that mental disorder is a Roschian concept. As Wakefield (1999: 377–8) shows, this argument fails. That a concept has vague boundaries is compatible with providing an account of it in terms of necessary and sufficient conditions. All that is needed is for at least one of the necessary and sufficient conditions to also be vague. Thus, to take Wakefield's example, it is vague whether an unmarried, sixteen-year-old male counts as a bachelor. Nonetheless, necessary and sufficient conditions for being a bachelor can be given. Someone is a bachelor if they are an unmarried adult male. Whether a particular individual is a bachelor can be vague because in some cases it may be vague whether they count as an adult.

Lilienfeld and Marino's only other reason for thinking that mental disorder is a Roschian concept is that attempts to provide necessary and sufficient conditions for the concept have repeatedly failed. In *Philosophical Investigations*, Wittgenstein concludes that "game" is a family resemblance term for similar reasons. Wittgenstein instructs us to "look and see whether there is anything common to all [games]" (Wittgenstein 1953: §66). Once we have seen that games have nothing in common we are led to conclude that "game" is a family resemblance concept. I suggest that the case of "mental disorder" is different. As we have seen, accounts that seek to provide necessary and sufficient conditions for something being a disorder are still being developed, and one of these accounts might yet prove to be adequate. As such, concluding that "disorder" is a family resemblance concept would be premature.

3.7 Conclusion

In this chapter I have provided an overview of current accounts of disorder. Table 3.1 summarizes the main accounts discussed, and the difficulties that they face.

As we have seen, there are currently several competing accounts of disease being developed, and it is not clear which, if any, will eventually prove satisfactory. There is much work still to be done with developing an account of disease. However, I suggest that a consensus is emerging with respect to some key issues: first, most of the accounts of disease being developed treat physical and mental disorders together. It is unlikely that the distinction between mental and physical disorder is of much importance. Secondly, there is a general consensus that diseases are necessarily harmful conditions. The prospects for purely descriptive accounts of disease (such as Boorse's) look bleak.

Some may worry that if disorder is a value-laden concept then the scientific status of psychiatry is thrown into doubt. I do not think this is a genuine concern. If disorder is a value-laden concept then this is important, but not that important. If disorders have to be bad states, and we assume that questions of value lie outside the realm of science, then determining whether a condition is a disorder is not a purely scientific issue. However, once the domain of disorders has been picked out, describing those disorders and working out how they are caused can be solely a matter for science. It is worth remembering that much scientific enquiry is directed at domains that are of interest to human beings because of the values that we have, so scientists look at food plants and agricultural pests, for example. Nonetheless, the truths that scientists discover about food plants, pests and mental disorders can be purely objective. To say that something is a pest involves values. But to say that it is black and shiny, and hibernates, does not. Similarly, even if saying that schizophrenia is a disorder involves values, claims about its typical characteristics and course need not.

Table 3.1 Summary of accounts of disorder

Account	Definition of disorders	Main difficulty
Boorse	Biological dysfunctions	Classifies homosexuality as a disorder. Cannot cope with the possibility that some disorders are biologically/ evolutionarily advantageous (and so not dysfunctions at all)
DSM/Wakefield	Harmful dysfunctions	Cannot cope with the possibility that some disorders are biologically/ evolutionarily advantageous (and so not dysfunctions at all)
Fulford	Illnesses are linked to failures in ordinary action. "Disease" is a family resemblance concept; diseases are linked to illnesses in a variety of ways	Are all disorders linked to failures of action? What of disfiguring conditions? Or those that produce abnormal sensations?
Aristotelian (Megone)	Incapacitating states that reduce flourishing	Fails to distinguish disorders from other types of bad state, such as certain non-disorder biological badness (e.g. ugliness), some social and educational bad states and vices.
Messy accounts (Reznek/ Cooper)	Harmful states that are potentially medically treatable. In addition Reznek adds that they must be abnormal. Cooper holds that the patient must be unlucky	Further work is needed to flesh out different criteria.
Roschian approaches	No necessary and sufficient criteria can be given	This is a "no-account account": an account of last resort

4. Explanations in psychiatry 1
Natural-history based explanations

In the previous two chapters we looked at the nature of mental disorder. We concluded that mental disorder is no myth. Furthermore, even if value judgements are involved in determining whether a condition is a disorder, projects that seek to investigate the causes and natural history of particular conditions can be properly scientific. With the subject matter of psychiatry assured, in this chapter and the next we shall consider the forms of explanation used in psychiatry. I focus particularly on two types of explanation that are frequently found in psychiatry but are less common in many other sciences. This chapter examines what I call "natural-history style explanations", and Chapter 5 examines how case histories function as explanations. At the outset it is worth noting that these are not the only forms of explanation found in psychiatry.[1] However, I focus on these particular types of explanation because they are characteristic of psychiatry and have been comparatively neglected by philosophers of science.

"Natural-history style" explanations work by invoking "natural kinds". "Natural kind" is a philosophical term of art, about which I shall have more to say later. For now we can say that paradigmatic examples of natural kinds are biological species and chemical elements. Such kinds are objective: it is a mind-independent fact about the world that lions and tigers are importantly different. They are also theoretically important: distinguishing between lions and tigers is important if one wants to conduct biological research. Members of a natural kind are plausibly naturally similar to each other because they are similar at a fundamental level. Tigers, for example, are all similar in that they are striped and have big teeth and eat meat, and tigers are alike in these respects because they are similar in some more fundamental way, for example, they all share a particular evolutionary history and are genetically similar.

"Natural-history style" explanations work in the following way. An individual is identified as being of a particular natural kind, say, a particular species, and its behaviour can then be explained and predicted; we can say that the individual will behave as things of its kind usually behave. For example, suppose I dig up potatoes only to find them riddled with holes. Eventually I find a potential culprit: a three-inch long, orange, multi-legged creature. There are several things I want to know. First, did this creature damage my potatoes, or did it just move into a hole caused by another: slugs maybe? Secondly, if it and others of its kind are eating my potatoes, how can I stop them? I look up the creature in a book and find that it is probably a spotted snake millipede. I discover that these millipedes like potatoes, they commonly enlarge holes caused by slugs, and there is nothing much I can do about them. The behaviour of the creature in my potato can now be explained and predicted. It is in my potato because it is eating it, it probably got in through a slug hole, and, if I do not kill it, it will eat more of my potatoes. This it what I mean by natural-history style explanation and prediction. Along similar lines, we can explain that Rex is likely to eat any meat left in his vicinity because that is what dogs do, that this raspberry is edible because all raspberries are edible, and that this piece of steel will be attracted to a magnet because all pieces of steel are attracted to magnets.

To summarize, paradigmatic examples of natural kinds are biological species and chemical elements. Such kinds are objective and theoretically important. Natural-history style explanations work by identifying the natural kind to which an individual belongs. Once the individual has been identified as being of a particular kind we can expect it to behave in the ways typical of its kind.

Those accustomed to the law-based explanations that are common in sciences such as physics may be tempted to look down on natural-history style explanations and predictions. This, however, would be a mistake. Admittedly, once we have a natural-history style explanation of an individual's behaviour there is still explanatory work to be done; if I say that Miffy is scared of dogs because she is a rabbit, then I may still want to go on to find an explanation of why it is that rabbits are in general scared of dogs. Still, natural-history style explanations and predictions can suffice for many purposes. Consider the successes of farmers, gardeners, herbalists, hunters and cooks. These are almost entirely based on natural-history style explanations and predictions. Thus the gardener can tell us that this seed needs to be planted in February because it is a broad bean, while another is a French bean and can wait until June. The cook knows that this mushroom can be eaten, but that another cannot. The farmer knows that this creature needs fresh greens to survive, but that another will make it through the winter on hay alone.

Natural history explanations can give us enormous power over the world. The explanations are admittedly incomplete, in so far as further explanatory work might tell us why all members of a kind behave as they do. Still, the explanations are sufficient for many purposes, and the predictions, of course, are perfectly acceptable predictions. The successes of natural-history style explanations and predictions are explicable in so far as we suppose that a particular classification mirrors real differences in the causal powers of entities in the world. Thus broad beans need to be planted in February and French beans in June because these different beans have distinct causal powers (grounded in properties that may as yet be unknown). Something about the constitution of broad beans means that they grow better if planted earlier in the year than French beans.[2]

Turning to psychiatry we can now see why it matters whether there are natural kinds of mental disorder. If there are natural kinds of disorder then we can hope for natural-history style explanations and predictions in psychiatry, and these might allow us to control and predict the course of disorders. Thus, the task of this chapter is to consider the role played by natural kinds and natural-history style explanations in psychiatry. At the outset it is worth noting that talk of natural kinds is not entirely foreign to psychiatry. Implicitly, much psychiatric practice assumes that many mental disorders can be expected to be natural kinds. Consider, for example, the assumptions that underpin the DSM (the classification of mental disorders produced by the APA): when revising the classification the relevant committees review thousands of empirical studies.[3] These empirical studies examine matters such as the biochemical correlates of disorders, how people with different disorders respond to particular treatments, and whether a particular disorder disproportionately affects people of a certain age or sex. In revising the DSM it is thus assumed that empirical research can tell us how mental disorders ought to be classified. The aim is to construct a classification system that at least approximately reflects the natural similarities and differences between cases of mental illness.

The similarities and differences between types of mental disease are assumed to be objective and also important for psychiatric theory. Psychiatric research generally focuses on groups of patients with the same diagnosis because these patients are assumed to be similar in some fundamental way. Implicitly, it is supposed that fundamentally different pathological processes underlie different disorders, and that different disorders are best treated in different ways.

At least implicitly, the APA aims to construct a classification system very much like those found in biology or chemistry. The differences between types of mental disorder are thought to be objective and theoretically important, in the same sort of way as are the differences between the chemical elements or biological species. The APA thus assumes that mental disorders are natural kinds.

In this chapter I argue that the assumption that types of mental disorder are natural kinds – an assumption that underpins much psychiatric theorizing and practice – is justified. There are plausibly natural kinds of mental disorder. This claim is controversial. Many theorists have claimed that mental disorders cannot be natural kinds and in the course of this chapter I shall have to show how their arguments fail. My argument that there are natural kinds in psychiatry will thus proceed in a somewhat roundabout way. I shall examine the reasons why many people have thought that there are not natural kinds in psychiatry, one by one, and show why each reason is inadequate. My argument that there are natural kinds of disorder then follows: there are plausible candidates for such kinds, and there is no good reason to deny them natural kind status.

4.1 More on natural kinds

4.1.1 Traditions distinguished

"Natural kind" is a technical philosophical term, but unfortunately it is used to mean different things by different writers. In this section I distinguish the sense in which I shall use "natural kind" from other possible senses. This section is chiefly included for those who have read something about natural kinds already, and who might be confused to find that I appear to be writing about something different. If you have never heard of natural kinds before, you will not need to know how the kinds I am writing of differ from other people's kinds, and can go straight to §4.1.2.

In the literature, one can find at least three fairly distinct groupings of people working on natural kinds. Each grouping uses "natural kind" in a somewhat different way.

- *Kinds-in-science tradition.* First, there are people who take natural kinds to be the kinds of thing, stuff or process studied by the natural sciences (e.g. Dupré 1993). Biological species and chemical elements are thus taken to be paradigmatic examples of natural kinds. In this tradition, natural kinds are supposed to be interesting because they feature in explanations, and can support inductive inferences. As philosophers working in this tradition need a label, and define natural kinds as being the kinds investigated by the natural sciences, I shall refer to them as the "kinds-in-science tradition". In the remainder of the chapter we shall be looking at "natural kinds" in this sense.
- *New essentialists.* As their name suggests, new essentialists like essences. The most famous of the new essentialists is Brian Ellis (2001; 2002). New essentialists think that there are some kinds where all members of the kind necessarily possess some identical "essential" property. For example, the essential property of gold would plausibly be having an atomic number of 79. That a sample of metal has an atomic number of 79 makes it gold, and also explains many of its properties: that the material has an atomic number of 79 explains why it is malleable, gold-coloured and inert. New essentialists explore the metaphysical consequences that might follow from kinds having essences. For example, some of them have claimed that the

existence of kinds that have essential properties implies that at least some physical laws are necessary.

Importantly, for the new essentialists only kinds that have essential properties count as natural kinds. Types of fundamental particle and chemical element are thus among the best candidates for being natural kinds. If other kinds, such as biological species, turn out not to have essential properties then, according to the new essentialists, they simply do not count as natural kinds. This stance sharply demarcates new essentialism from the kinds-in-science tradition. In the kinds-in-science tradition, as we have seen, biological species are taken to be paradigmatic examples of natural kinds.

- *Aristotelians.* Aristotelian approaches to natural kinds will be familiar to some readers interested in the philosophy of psychiatry through Megone's (1998) writings. Aristotelians are somewhat like new essentialists in that they claim that natural kinds possess essential properties. However, the sorts of properties that Aristotelians and new essentialists consider to be suitable candidates for being essences are very different. As we saw, when pushed to give examples, new essentialists will probably nominate properties such as atomic numbers as plausible candidates for being essential properties. In contrast an Aristotelian is more likely to offer biological species as paradigmatic examples of natural kinds, and will suggest, for example, that the essential property of being human is "being a rational animal". Aristotelians emphasize how the members of different natural kinds can be expected to go through different characteristic life cycles. They claim that the essential property of the kind ensures that its members develop as they should. Both Aristotelians and new essentialists think that the essential property possessed by a member of a kind causes it to have many of the other properties that it has. So, while a new essentialist will say that having an atomic number of 79 explains why gold has certain features, an Aristotelian will say that it is because human beings are rational animals that they can use language, laugh and so on. That the Aristotelian and new essentialist nominate very different properties as candidates for being essential properties stems from their very different notions of causation. Despite the fact that both Aristotelians and new essentialists think that natural kinds possess essential properties, their deeper metaphysical differences (about the nature of causation and explanation, for example) mean that new essentialists and Aristotelians belong to very different traditions.

When philosophers working in these different traditions talk to each other they tend to talk at cross purposes. In the different traditions people use "natural kind" in different ways, and are interested in different questions. The traditions even disagree as to what might count as paradigmatic examples of natural kinds. Thus, new essentialists consider physical particles to be paradigmatic examples of natural kinds and are dubious about biological species, while Aristotelians take the exact opposite line. Doubtless, if one were to look into the histories of the debates on natural kinds in sufficient detail there will turn out to be deep and interesting connections between them. Exploring such connections would be a task for another time, however. To a first approximation at least, these different debates are simply distinct, and "natural kind" is used in a slightly different way in each. Thus, if one wants to avoid confusion, when talking about natural kinds the best strategy is to state at the outset how one is defining "natural kind".

In this chapter I examine whether types of mental disorders are natural kinds in the sense of the "kinds-in-science" tradition. New essentialist and Aristotelian conceptions of natural kinds will henceforth be ignored in this chapter. This is not because new essentialist or Aristotelian approaches to kinds are unimportant, but simply because they are not what I am dealing with here. I shall take it that "natural kinds" are paradigmatically the kinds picked out by the natural sciences. These kinds feature in laws and can ground explanations and sound inductive inferences. The task here is to examine whether mental disorders can be considered to be kinds in such a sense.

4.1.2 Accounts of natural kinds

The task of this chapter is to find out whether types of mental disorder can be considered natural kinds in the sense in which biological species and chemical elements are natural kinds. This question is important because of the links such kinds have with explanations, laws and inductive inferences.[4] First, however, we must seek a philosophical account of such kinds. How is it that natural kinds can feature in explanations and laws and support sound inductive inferences?

One initially attractive account will not quite do. It is tempting to think that all members of a natural kind behave similarly because they are essentially all the same: there is some essential property that determines their other properties. Such an account will not do for biological species because it is plausible that there is no essential property that all members of a species share. As John Dupré (1981: 84–5) has pointed out, there are reasons for thinking that often there will be no one genetic property or set of properties shared by all members of a species: evolutionary theory leads us to expect there will be variation in the genes possessed by members of a species. Genetic disorders and mutations also mean that the genetic properties of members of a kind will vary.

As mentioned previously, new essentialists respond to such difficulties by arguing that if biological species lack essential properties then this only goes to show that they are not natural kinds. They then stop thinking about kinds such as biological species. Here we will not take this route. We need to understand how kinds such as biological species can play the role in science that they do. This is because mental disorders can be expected to be more like other biological kinds than like the kinds found in fundamental physics and chemistry. As such we must understand how biological species support laws, explanations and inductive inferences if we are to see whether and how types of mental disorder can do similar work.

This way of thinking goes against some recent writings in the philosophy of psychiatry. Peter Zachar (2000) accepts that natural kinds must have essences, and thus holds that neither biological species nor mental disorders can be natural kinds. He suggests that both mental disorders and biological species should instead be thought of as what he calls "practical kinds", which are kinds that it is useful to pick out for some purposes. The problem with such an approach becomes apparent once we ask why it is that some "practical kinds" can better serve as the basis for explanations and predictions than others. Kinds such as "tiger" provide a better basis for explanations and predictions than do kinds such as "drug" (Zachar's example of a practical kind). There are many generalizations that we can make about tigers ("Tigers are stripy", "Tigers eat meat", "Tigers are not native to the UK"). In contrast there are very few generalizations that we can make about "drugs". "Drug" is sometimes defined as being a substance that alters the functioning of an organism, but beyond this drugs have little in common. It is not even true that all drugs can be found in pharmacies, as pharmacies do not sell crack cocaine. If we want to know why "tiger" is a better kind than "drug" we will be forced into developing an account of how it is that kinds such as biological species can support laws, explanations and inductive inferences while many other kinds cannot. Kinds such as biological species are better kinds than many "practical kinds". Our project is to understand why this is the case, and then to consider whether kinds of mental disorder can plausibly be expected to support explanations and predictions in the same sorts of way.

Various accounts of natural kinds have been developed that can accommodate biological species. As it is plausible that biological species lack essential properties, these are all non-essentialist accounts, that is, they are accounts of natural kinds that do not claim that all members of a kind share some *identical* essential property. Instead they claim that biological species are natural kinds because their members are objectively *similar* to each other in ways that are theoretically important. For example, Dupré (1981; 1993) argues for an account he calls "promiscuous realism". He asks us to imagine the individual entities of some domain mapped out on a multidimensional quality space (that is a multidimensional graph where the dimensions correspond to different qualities). In such a space, two entities with identical properties, such as two identical ladybirds, end up at the same point. On the other hand, two entities with very different properties, such as a ladybird and an elephant, end up far from each other on the graph. Dupré claims that, if we plotted the entities in the world onto a multidimensional quality space, we would find numerous clusters corresponding to groups of similar entities.

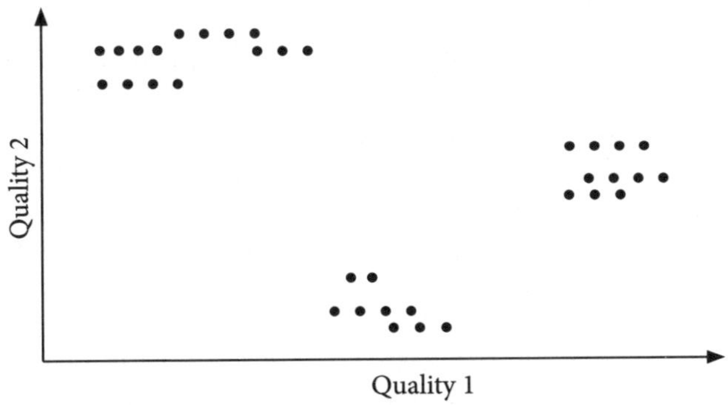

Figure 4.1 Two dimensions of a multidimensional quality space, showing three clusters of similar entities.

On Dupré's account, some clusters will be formed by the members of traditional natural kinds. There will be clusters of dogs, cats and dandelions, for example. At different levels of resolution it will also be possible to make out other clusters. Not only will there be a cluster that corresponds to dogs, but at finer levels there will also be clusters that correspond to Border Collies and to Alsatians, and at still finer levels there may be clusters that correspond to the dogs that make up a particular pedigree. In many cases the clusters will not be discrete, but will be messy and hard to make out. Different clusters can also be generated by restricting our attention to particular dimensions of the map. If we focus on the dimensions that code for nutritional value, for example, we will find a cluster of things that are poisonous to human beings. Dupré's account is realist because the clusters in quality space reflect the real structure of nature. It is promiscuous because there will be many different clusters on which we could choose to focus. On Dupré's account the members of a species will cluster together in the multidimensional property space because they are similar to each other in a variety of ways. As the members of the kind are similar to each other they can be expected to behave in similar ways.

Here, in an account inspired by Dupré, when we ask whether types of mental disorder are natural kinds, we will count types of mental disorder as natural kinds if they meet the following conditions:

- all cases of the disorder are similar in theoretically important ways; and
- these similarities are objective, that is, they do not simply depend on the observer.

It is worth noting that paradigmatic examples of natural kinds meet these requirements. All samples of a chemical element, and all members of a biological species, are objectively similar to each other in theoretically important ways. Conversely many kinds fail to be natural kinds on this account. Thus, the kind "things on Rachel's desk" fails to be a natural kind because the things on my desk are motley: they fail to be objectively similar to each other in theoretically important ways.

Clearly, this is a very minimal account of natural kinds. However, it is sufficient for our purposes. If any mental disorder meets these requirements then that will be enough to explain how it is that saying that a particular case is of that type can function as an explanation, and also to ground predictions about the course of the disorder. If all cases of a disorder are similar in objective and theoretically important ways then they can be expected to behave similarly to each other.

It is worth reiterating that we are not here committed to essentialism; on our non-essentialist account members of a natural kind need only be objectively similar in theoretically important ways – they do not have to be fundamentally identical.

Often authors have claimed that natural kinds must be discrete. In other words, they have held that any two kinds have natural boundaries between them and that intermediate forms do not occur (e.g. Mill [1843] 1973: 123; De Sousa 1984: 565; Haslam 2002). This is a claim that tends to be assumed rather than argued for, and I see no reason to make it. It is the fact that members of a natural kind are similar that does all the work when it comes to making inductive inferences and grounding explanations. It is because members of a natural kind all have similar properties that we can predict that all members of a natural kind will behave similarly. As the "gaps" between natural kinds do no metaphysical work, there seems to be no reason to claim that natural kinds must be discrete. In addition, abandoning the discreteness claim has the advantage that kinds that are not discrete, such as alloys, can be accommodated within a natural kind account. Taking alloys to be natural kinds seems to me justifiable because knowing that a sample is a particular alloy is as useful, and useful in the same kinds of ways, as knowing that it is a 100 per cent pure metal. If a sample is known to be fifty-five per cent zinc and forty-five per cent copper, one can predict how the sample will behave just as well as if one knew it to be pure copper. We should thus allow that some natural kind domains may be continuous. So, if depression turns out to be continuous with anxiety, say, then depression can still be a natural kind on our account. All that is required is that all cases of depression are objectively similar to each other in theoretically important ways.

4.2 Arguments against mental disorders being natural kinds

Various writers have argued that types of mental disorder cannot be natural kinds. Most of their arguments have sought to show that mental disorders cannot be natural kinds on a traditional, essentialist understanding of natural kind. We are using a weaker notion of natural kind. Nevertheless, if the arguments considered here worked, they would also show that mental disorders could not be natural kinds on our account of natural kinds. As such, in this section I examine the arguments one by one, and seek to show why they fail.

4.2.1 The variation objection

One reason that leads people to doubt that there can be natural kinds of mental disorder is that types of mental disorder have varied greatly across cultures and history. To many this makes it look as if kinds of objectively similar cases of disorder cannot be picked out: the disorders that are found in one context are simply different from those found in another. A plausible corollary of such a view would be that mental disorders can only be understood via ideographic as opposed to nomothetic means (i.e. they would need to be understood via historical case studies instead of via a law-based science).

In this section I shall first present examples that show that some mental disorders plausibly do differ at different times and in different places. Then, secondly, I shall argue that such disorders might nevertheless be natural kinds.

As an example of the ways in which disorders can be shaped by cultural context consider this case from Richard Freiherr von Krafft-Ebing's *Psychopathia Sexualis* (first published in German in 1886). Krafft-Ebing's Case 129 concerns a man who would nowadays be considered transsexual. He says, "I feel like a woman in a man's form; and even though I often am sensible of the man's form, yet it is always in a feminine sense. Thus, for example, I feel the penis as a clitoris" ([1886] 1998: 207). The patient then goes on to make statements that clearly suggest that feelings of "being trapped in the wrong body" can be culturally shaped. For example, the patient knows he is really a woman because, "I have the sensations of a woman. I cannot go with bare hands, as both heat and cold trouble me" (*ibid.*). He "could not endure obscenity" (*ibid.*: 203), and has problems wearing trousers as his female abdomen cannot stand the pressure. Worst of all, while the patient previously perspired little, "now there are all the odious peculiarities of the female perspiration, particularly about the lower part of the body" (*ibid.*: 206). Here the patient's beliefs about women – that, for example, they are sensitive, sweaty and oddly allergic to swear words – clearly affect the sensations that he experiences. With a change in cultural beliefs the symptoms experienced by transsexuals have plausibly altered.

For our second example we will go further back and take a case that will be familiar to philosophers. In *The Meditations* Descartes considers whether his sense perceptions might be mistaken. At one point he wonders whether he might be insane. In particular he wonders whether he might be one of:

> those insane persons whose minds are so troubled and clouded by the black vapours of the bile that they constantly assert that they are kings, when they are very poor; that they are wearing gold and purple, when they are quite naked; or who imagine that they are pitchers or that they have a body of glass. ([1641] 1968: 96)

People who have delusions of grandeur and, for example, believe they are kings, are still found today. People who think they have bodies of glass are no longer seen. However, during the early modern period, Glass and Earthenware Men were relatively commonplace. In her study of the glass delusion in Europe between 1440 and 1680, Gill Speak (1990) describes numerous cases. In 1561, for example, Lemnius described a patient who believed himself to have glass buttocks and was thus afraid of shattering if he sat down (Lemnius notes that this patient could only relieve himself standing up). Around 1614, Alfonso Ponce de Santa Cruze reports on a Glass Man who was afraid of breaking and took to a straw bed at his physician's suggestion. Applying unconventional therapy, "a conveniently arranged fire restored him to his senses". Speak notes that Glass Men also featured prominently in the literature of the time. The glass delusion was once a paradigmatic example of insanity, but is not seen today. Speak considers that the glass delusion reflected religious themes on the fragility and transience of life. In a less pious time, such themes touch us less, and nowadays other delusions are found.

The examples of Krafft-Ebing's transsexual and the Glass Men show that mental disorders vary with context. As mentioned earlier, many assume that where there is variation there cannot be natural kinds. Thus, Stephan Fuchs (2001) states: "Natural kinds always exist, or seem to exist, independent of relationships, context, time, or observer". He goes on: "Allowing for variation means dissolving natural kinds" (*ibid.*: 13). Still, although many have thought that variation is incompatible with the existence of natural kinds, this view is incorrect. Variation is in fact consistent with there being natural kinds of mental disorder, for two reasons: the existence of ecological niches and the fact that the characteristics of natural kinds may vary with environmental conditions.

First response: ecological niches

The idea that mental disorders may require a particular "ecological niche" to exist is best developed by Ian Hacking in his book *Mad Travelers* (1998). In *Mad Travelers* Hacking uses fugue as a case study to examine why it is that some mental disorders appear to thrive only at a particular place and time, or to be, as he puts it, "transient". Fugue was a dissociative disorder characterized by travel and amnesia. Those who suffered from fugue felt compelled to wander, and suffered from altered states of consciousness. They would come to, many miles from home, with no idea what they were doing. Hacking claims that fugue, as a significant mental disorder, existed only in France between 1887 and 1909 (although, as we shall see shortly, the accuracy of this claim may be disputed).

Hacking's key contribution to understanding transient mental disorders is his metaphor of the ecological niche. Like biological organisms, Hacking suggests, transient mental disorders can only flourish within a particular environment. While organisms depend on food supplies and breeding sites, mental disorders thrive with a medical community that will recognize them, and a contemporary culture that creates space for them between healthy, virtuous activities on the one hand, and vicious, criminal ones on the other. According to Hacking, in the 1890s France provided the perfect environment for fugue. Police controls meant that wandering men would soon be picked up, and the medical community was happy to recognize fugue as a sub-type of either epilepsy or hysteria. At the same time cultural fascination with tourism and vagrancy allowed fugue to thrive in the ambiguous space between.

Hacking's idea that a disease may need an ecological niche makes good sense (although one might take issue with some of the factors that he thinks are needed for a niche). It is undeniable that many physical disorders only flourish within a particular social environment: if people did not keep pigeons there would be no pigeon fancier's lung; without asbestos there can be no asbestosis. It is plausible that mental disorders may also require specific environments.

I have some reservations about Hacking's use of fugue as an example of a transient mental disorder. Hacking claims that fugue, as a significant mental disorder, existed only in France between 1887 and 1909. He notes that fugue has been included in the DSM since 1980 but dismisses this as the result of political wangling by the proponents of multiple personality disorder (since both fugue and multiple personality disorder are classed as dissociative disorders the inclusion of one strengthens the case for the inclusion of the other). I question Hacking's claim that fugue died in 1909. Fugue was included as a diagnosis in the first DSM, published in 1952, and in its predecessor, the *Statistical Manual for the Use of Hospitals for Mental Diseases* (National Committee for Mental Hygiene 1945). Its inclusion in these taxonomies cannot be attributed to the 1970s and 1980s fights over multiple personality disorder. Moreover, the current DSM (1994) estimates that today 0.2 per cent of the general population meet the criteria for fugue; this compares with 0.2–2 per cent for schizophrenia. If these figures are correct then fugue is a fairly rare disorder, but still very much alive and kicking.

Still, we do not need to buy into Hacking's particular claims about fugue and its ecological niche to see that he is right in saying that mental disorders can be perfectly real and yet not found everywhere. Indeed, it is quite normal for members of a natural kind to be found only in certain places and at certain times, because they can exist only under certain conditions: pandas are found only where there is bamboo; house martins will live only where there are suitable nesting sites. There are also non-biological examples of kinds that are found only in particular environments. Many radioactive elements can be artificially manufactured but are not found naturally. Such elements are perfectly good natural kinds, but their half-lives are so short that the quantities of element created early in the history of the universe have long ago decayed. Differing environmental conditions mean that members of a kind are found in some places but not in others.

Similarly, Hacking is correct in claiming that kinds of mental disorder may require particular environments. The most obvious examples are disorders caused by nutritional deficiencies, poisons or drugs. Where there is no heroin there are no heroin addicts. Where people's diet contains sufficient iodine, cretinism is rare. Such examples may be too "biological" for some readers. However, more purely psychological kinds may also require particular environments. Post traumatic stress disorder is caused by trauma. There is thus more of it where there are wars or natural disasters, and less of it where people's lives tend to pass peacefully.

Second response: Variation is permitted

Another response to the variation objection is to point out that the superficial properties of even non-controversial natural kinds commonly vary with environment. Thus, the tomatoes in my greenhouse grow bigger and quicker than those outside because of the extra warmth, and animals regularly have thicker fur in colder climates. As a consequence of such effects, members of the same natural kind can look different in different conditions.

The superficial properties of kinds of mental disorder may also vary with environment. In the West, depression is commonplace. In China, patients are more likely to complain of symptoms such as fatigue, pains and sleep disturbance, and are diagnosed as suffering from neurasthenia. Nonetheless, some theorists think that the condition that underlies both neurasthenia and depression will turn out to be the same (Parker *et al.* 2001). Or, as we have seen, the content of typical delusions changes over time. While deluded people once thought they were made of glass, now they fear radioactive contamination. Still, while the content shifts, the underlying cause of the delusions may remain constant.

I conclude that, as the incidence and superficial properties of members of a kind commonly vary with environment, the perceived variation in human psychology is compatible with there being natural kinds of mental disorder.

4.2.2 Hacking's looping objection

Hacking's looping objection can be seen as a sophisticated version of the variation objection. In a series of papers written between 1986 and 1995, Hacking (1986, 1988, 1992, 1995a, 1995b) argued that what he calls "human kinds" cannot be natural kinds. Hacking's human kinds are the kinds distinguished by the human sciences, and would include any kinds of mental disorder. Hacking argues that human kinds are commonly altered by "looping effects" that occur when people change their behaviour in response to the ways in which they are classified. Thus obese people, for example, will know that they are considered obese and that obesity is stigmatized. This may well lead to changes in their behaviour: they may spend time trying to lose weight; they may resist and join the Fat Pride movement; they may get their stomachs stabled. In any event, there is "feedback" between the classification and the people being classified. Such looping results in human kinds having histories unlike prototypical natural kinds, leading Hacking to conclude that human kinds cannot be natural kinds.

More recently Hacking seems to have changed his mind and, although he never explicitly abandons his old argument, in *The Social Construction of What?* (1999) he discusses the possibility that at least some mental disorders might be natural kinds. My task here is to refute arguments that mental disorders cannot be natural kinds, so I shall only be concerned with Hacking's earlier work.

In his earlier series of papers Hacking presents us with detailed case studies that show how the behaviour typical of a human kind evolves hand in hand with the descriptions of it. I accept that feedback occurs when human kinds are classified, as Hacking describes. However, I argue that Hacking's claim that such histories show that human kinds cannot be natural kinds is false. My starting-point is that we should remember that our classificatory practices also result in feedback that alters some natural kinds (Bogen 1988). For example, the characteristics of domestic livestock change over time because particular animals are classified as being the "best in show" and are used in selective breeding. So the occurrence of feedback does not distinguish human kinds from natural kinds.

When faced with such examples, Hacking claims that the feedback that affects human kinds is importantly different from other types of feedback because it occurs as a result of subjects becoming *aware* of the ways in which they are being described and judged (Hacking 1997: 15). This idea needs working on before it can become an argument that human kinds cannot be natural kinds. Why does Hacking think that feedback that occurs as a result of subjects' ideas is metaphysically significant in a way that feedback caused by, say, selective breeding is not?

One might think that idea-dependence matters because it indicates that a kind is subjective. Then the argument would be that while natural kinds are objective, human kinds are affected by ideas and so are subjective, and that thus human kinds cannot be natural kinds. This is not a line of argument that Hacking himself pursues. Still, it is the most obvious route for someone who wishes to claim that idea-dependence is metaphysically significant and so worth exploring here.

At this point, however, we should note that entities can be idea-dependent in fundamentally different senses, not all of which are indicative of subjectivity.

Beauty, they say, is in the eye of the beholder. Indeed, it is easy to imagine that a woman wearing ornate false eyelashes may appear beautiful one year and absurd the next, depending on the whims of fashion. In this case the "change" from beautiful to absurd is a relational change only: it is brought about by a change in the viewer rather than by a change in the woman. Such idea-dependence indeed shows that a kind, such as beautiful women, is subjective and thus cannot be a natural kind.

But there is also another sort of idea-dependence. Imagine that the woman starts wearing false eyelashes because she reads that they are this season's essential accessory. Here ideas regarding beauty have affected her. They are part of the causal story that culminates in her wearing false eyelashes. However, the resulting change is perfectly objective. She used not to wear false eyelashes; now she does. Idea-dependence of this causal type results in objective changes in entities and is compatible with a kind, such as women who wear false eyelashes, being objective. Indeed, there might be interesting laws concerning such kinds, for example, conceivably, "Women who wear false eyelashes are more likely to get eye infections".

Hacking has shown that human kinds are affected by ideas. In order to show that human kinds are subjective he also needs to show that human kinds are affected by ideas in a way that results in relational as opposed to genuine changes. Hacking's examples, however, appear to be of cases where ideas produce genuine changes in peoples' behaviour. His most detailed case study concerns multiple personality disorder (Hacking 1995a). The first patients diagnosed with multiple personality disorder tended to have only two or three different personalities. As time passed more and more flamboyant cases started to appear on American chat shows; these patients had scores of different personalities, personalities of the opposite sex and animal personalities. Hacking argues that as a result more and more patients started presenting with similar symptoms. Popular ideas about multiple personality disorder affected the symptoms typical of patients. Nonetheless, it seems that the changes in patients' symptoms were genuine; patients really did start talking in a multitude of voices, for example. In order to show that the changes in the symptoms of multiple personality disorder indicate that it is a subjective kind and so not a natural kind Hacking would need to show that the changes in symptoms were not genuine, and he makes no suggestion that this is the case. Thus, I conclude that Hacking's argument has failed to show that types of mental disorder cannot be natural kinds.

In addition to the argument concerning feedback considered here, Hacking also offers another argument that mental disorders cannot be natural kinds. This argument centres on the idea that intentional actions are only intentional under certain descriptions, and that therefore new descriptions of possible actions (i.e. as produced by the human sciences) make new intentional actions possible (Hacking 1986). Hacking himself seems to put less weight on this argument (in that he presents it less frequently), it gets complicated and I have argued elsewhere that it does not work (Cooper 2004); for these reasons Hacking's second argument will not be discussed here.

4.2.3 The functionalist's objection

The objection

In "Mental States, Natural Kinds and Psychophysical Laws", Colin McGinn (1991) argues that if a functionalist account of mind is adopted, mental or psychological kinds cannot be considered natural kinds.[5] If he is correct, then in so far as functionalism is an attractive account of mind, it looks as if types of mental disorder cannot be natural kinds.

Functionalists hold that for something to count as a particular mental state it just has to play an appropriate functional role. The functional role that is appropriate for a particular mental state is characterized in terms of its typical sensory causes, typical behavioural effects and typical interactions with other mental states. So, to take an example, let us consider how a functionalist would characterize my belief that the dog coming towards me is dangerous. Such beliefs have the following causal role:

- they are typically caused by seeing dogs that are big and growling;
- they typically lead to avoidance behaviour such as crossing the road; and
- they typically cause other mental states such as fear, and then relief when I have moved past the dog.

In my case, my belief that the dog is dangerous will be realized by some neural activity. However, according to the functionalist there may also be beings that are physically very unlike me but that share my belief about the dog. For the functionalist *any* state that plays the right functional role – that is caused by seeing growling, and leads to avoidance behaviour and fear – will also count as having a belief that the dog is dangerous. The question of how the belief is physically realized is unimportant; all that matters is that the belief occupies the right functional role. So, a robot might share my belief about the dog even though the robot has no brain, and in its case the belief is realized by electronic gadgetry. That the same mental state can be realized by multiple physical, or even possibly non-physical, systems is called *multiple realizability*. Multiple realization implies that instances of a mental state can be physically dissimilar.

The functionalist claims that kinds of mental state are functionally defined kinds (i.e. they are defined in terms of their functional role). Other examples of functionally defined kinds are mousetraps and computer programs. For something to be a mousetrap it just has to catch mice; it does not matter what it is made from. Similarly, computer programs are defined in terms of their functional role. All functionally defined kinds are multiply realizable: instances of the kind can be made from physically different materials.

McGinn holds that multiple realization means that functionally defined kinds are importantly different from prototypical natural kinds. Members of prototypical natural kinds, such as chemical elements and biological species, are physically similar. So, all samples of an element share the same atomic number, and all tigers are genetically similar, for example. In contrast, members of functionally defined kinds can be physically diverse. Thus, while prototypical natural kinds can be characterized in terms of the similar physical properties that their members all possess, this will not work for functionally defined kinds.

Although members of a functionally defined kind can differ physically, all members of the kind have to be able to fulfil the same functional role. What, then, of the possibility that members of a psychological state just have their similar causal roles in common and that this is enough to count them as natural kinds? McGinn gives three reasons for rejecting this move.

First, McGinn claims that there will be no particular causal role that can be taken to be characteristic of a type of mental state. This is because mental states operate *holistically*. This means that what a particular mental state does varies with the other mental states possessed by the agent. So, once you know I am afraid of the dog, you cannot simply conclude that I will cross the road to avoid it. Maybe I am trying to put on a show of bravery, and so I will keep to the path that I am on. Maybe, I am afraid for my own safety, but even more concerned about the small old lady who is walking the dangerous dog, and so I offer to take it from her. What a mental state does depends radically on circumstances. As such, McGinn concludes that there may well be no particular causal role that can be used to identify a mental state.

Secondly, McGinn draws our attention to the fact that the properties that make members of paradigmatic natural kinds similar have to do with their internal constitution. Functionally defined properties are different because they are specifically not linked to the internal constitution of entities.

Thirdly, McGinn claims that any specification of a mental state's causal role would be true by definition rather than an empirical discovery. It is not an empirical discovery that those who want chocolate seek chocolate; this is part of what it means to want chocolate! In contrast, finding out which properties characterize prototypical natural kinds takes empirical work. Scientists had to do research to discover that all samples of gold have an atomic number of 79, or that water is H_2O.

Functionalism is an attractive view of the mind. If functionalism is correct, then multiple realizability means that psychological kinds cannot be characterized in terms of shared physical properties. The only other option would be to try to define psychological kinds in terms of functionally defined properties.

However, McGinn claims, kinds characterized by functionally defined properties would differ so radically from prototypical natural kinds that they should not be considered natural kinds at all. It follows, he thinks, that if functionalism is correct, then psychological kinds cannot be natural kinds.

A response

Multiple realization causes problems for the idea that psychological kinds are natural kinds because it means that mental states of the same type can be physically diverse. Dreams of characterizing pain in terms of C-fibre activation, or some such, will be unachievable if Martians and robots can be in pain but lack all C-fibres.

Plausibly, though, there is a way of dealing with such problems. Multiple realization means that instances of pain may be physically diverse; my pain may have nothing physically in common with that of an octopus or an alien. Nevertheless, instances of *normal human* pain may all be physically alike (Kim 1993: 309–35). Indeed, there are reasons for thinking this is likely to be the case. Painkillers are effective, and they do not work by magic or by reprogramming our software. Rather, they must work by interacting with the physical properties that underlie pain in normal human beings. The functionalist claims that pain might be realized by all sorts of odd physical systems. But they can consistently also think that instances of normal human pain may well be physically alike, and indeed may form a natural kind.

This being said we should accept that there may be unusual human beings who for some reason or other realize pain differently. And, indeed, it might turn out that there are various different sorts of normal human pain, in the same sort of way that there are different varieties of normal human blood. If this turned out to be the case, then further retreat would be required, and normal human pain might be divided into a number of physically different sub-types – pain A, pain B, pain C and so on – but of course these could themselves constitute different natural kinds.

A functionalist can consistently hold that normal human pain might turn out to be one natural kind or a number of different natural kinds. Other sorts of normal human mental state might similarly fall into natural kinds. There might be natural kinds of normal human emotion or normal human sensation, for example. In such cases one can imagine that future scientific evidence might show that instances of the normal human mental state are physically similar. Maybe all feelings of disgust or depression, or all tickling sensations, will be linked with a particular type of neural activity.

As we can see from these examples, two of McGinn's concerns can easily be dealt with. Suppose that cases of human depression can be characterized by an abnormality in neurotransmitter levels. Then all cases of depression in human beings will be physically similar. In addition, as McGinn demands, the nature of depression would have been discovered empirically, rather than being true by definition.

Only McGinn's concern about the holism of the mental remains as a worry. Here it will help to distinguish between propositional and non-propositional mental states. Propositional states are those with content: they are characterized in terms of what they are about. Examples are: "I believe that Paris is in France"; "I hope that my plane will be on time"; and "I fear that my croissant is stale". In contrast, non-propositional mental states are not straightforwardly about anything. Propositional mental states operate holistically, and as a consequence they cannot be matched up with a characteristic causal role. However, McGinn has overlooked the fact that at least some non-propositional mental states are different. Some non-propositional mental states do tend to produce characteristic effects regardless of an agent's other mental states. So, if I am in a lot of pain I will tend to swear, cry or scream. In certain situations I may suppress these behaviours, but the urge to express my pain will still be there, it will just be held back by other forces (I will have to bite my lip to hold back my tears). That the characteristic effects of pain can be suppressed makes it no different from most physical happenings. Gravity tends to make apples fall, although some apples may be caught. Similarly, being in pain tends to produce crying, although some crying is suppressed. At least some non-propositional mental states do not operate holistically, and will not be affected by McGinn's argument.

So one can be a sort of functionalist and yet hold that at least some human psychological kinds are natural kinds. When Martians feel pain or fear, these states might be realized in all sorts of odd ways. Nevertheless, instances of some mental states in human beings might be physically alike, and such psychological kinds in human beings might be natural kinds. And, among other psychological kinds, there might be natural kinds of mental disorder.

4.3 Are types of mental disorder natural kinds?

I have shown that arguments that types of mental disorder cannot be natural kinds fail. Before going on to the positive argument, and considering whether it is likely that any types of mental disorder actually are natural kinds, one last difficulty must be dealt with. Thus far all the examples of natural kinds we have considered have been types of thing or stuff. Types of mental disorder should not be thought of in this way but should instead in general be thought of as types of process. A major depressive episode, for example, has a beginning, progresses and then ends.

That mental disorders are often best thought of as processes is not a big problem, as accounts of natural kinds can be readily adapted to deal with natural kinds of process. One can say that instances of a natural kind of process will all be fundamentally similar to each other *so long as they are at the same stage.* Types of disease will not be the only sort of natural kinds of process. Other examples might be particular chemical reactions, for example, rusting, and particular biological processes, for example, the metamorphosis of some particular species of caterpillar into a butterfly.

On our modest construal of "natural kind", for types of mental disorder to be natural kinds it must be the case that instances of the disorder are all similar to each other in some fundamental sense. Unfortunately many mental disorders are insufficiently well understood for it to be possible to know whether or not this criterion is met. Plausibly, however, there are at least some mental disorders that meet this condition. Huntington's disease seems to be a likely example. This disorder is caused by a single dominant gene on chromosome four. Symptoms normally appear in middle-age and include jerky involuntary movements, behavioural changes and progressive dementia. Huntington's disease is plausibly a natural kind of mental disorder; in all instances an identical underlying property, the defective gene, produces characteristic symptoms. Other mental disorders that would count as natural kinds on my account would be any where it turned out that all cases shared some particular imbalance of neurotransmitters, for example.

Some types of mental disorder are plausibly natural kinds. However, there will also be cases where current diagnoses group together cases that do not share any theoretically important features and do not form natural kinds. "Rag-bag" diagnoses that are given codes in the DSM such as "psychotic disorder not otherwise specified" are the most obvious examples here. Moreover, future research may eventually show that some better entrenched diagnoses also turn out not to group together natural kinds. Some suggest that this is likely to be the case with schizophrenia, for example.[6]

4.4 Consequences

I have argued that some mental disorders are plausibly natural kinds. At this point it is worth reminding ourselves why this would matter. The main reason why it is important is that if mental disorders are natural kinds we may then hope for natural-history style explanations and predictions in psychiatry. If bipolar disorder, say, turns out to be a natural kind, then we can explain why it is that a particular case unfolds as it does. We can say that someone suffers from alternating manic and depressive phases *because* they have bipolar disorder. We will also be able to make various predictions, for example, if someone suffers from bipolar disorder then lithium treatment might help. Where mental disorders are natural kinds, this will give us some control over them. In particular, treatments that work for one of the kind can be expected to work for all of the kind.

Before the end of this chapter, a little should be said about the potential ethical and political implications of holding that some types of mental disorder are natural kinds. Some link the claim that there are natural kinds in psychiatry or psychology to reactionary political beliefs. For example, in *The Disorder of Things*, Dupré writes that when types of people are considered to form distinct natural kinds "it is inevitable that any systematic differences that are found will be taken to be explained, or explicable, in terms of the intrinsic differences between members of the two kinds" (Dupré 1993: 253). This leads to the "legitimation of conservative politics and to the discouragement of proposals for significant social change" (*ibid*.: 256). Dupré's thought appears to be that if some disadvantaged group form a natural kind then their state is natural and thus unalterable.

Dupré's worry can be responded to in two ways. First, we must remember that the world is often not as we would like it to be. Even if unfortunate political implications were to follow, this does not show that there are no natural kinds in psychiatry. Ethics cannot drive metaphysics. Secondly, and along more conciliatory lines, at least on the modest construal of natural kind that is in play here, the political implications of there being natural kinds of mental disorder are far more limited than Dupré suggests. The members of a natural kind can be destroyed. Moreover, the superficial properties of natural kinds commonly vary with environment, and so can be changed by altering the environment. So, let us suppose that heroin addicts form a natural kind. Heroin affects the brains and bodies of heroin addicts producing characteristic effects. Nevertheless, heroin addicts can stop taking the drug and cease to be members of the natural kind. While addicted to heroin, their brains are a certain way, and they are members of the kind "heroin addict", but when addicts stop taking heroin, their brains recover, and they cease to be members of the kind. Furthermore, even if heroin addiction is a natural kind, the characteristics of being a heroin addict can vary with environment. When clean needles and purer drugs are available, the consequences of being an addict will be less severe than in other environments, for example. Thus, one can consistently hold that some disadvantaged group form a natural kind, and also think that their situation could be improved by social changes.

4.5 Conclusion

To summarize, in this chapter we have seen that different philosophical traditions have different understandings of "natural kind". For our purposes we took it that types of mental disorder would be natural kinds if cases of the disorder are objectively similar in theoretically important ways. On such an account we are not committed to essentialism. Nor are we committed to discreteness (there need not be gaps between natural kinds).

We looked at popular arguments that mental disorders are not natural kinds, and saw that they fail. First, mental disorders can be natural kinds despite the variation that is seen across times and cultures, as natural kinds commonly need particular ecological niches to survive, and the superficial characteristics of natural kinds often vary with environment. Secondly, mental disorders can be natural kinds despite Hacking's argument that subjects are affected by the ways in which they are classified. The members of some natural kinds are also affected by our classifications, and for ideas to feature in the causal history that leads to a kind having particular characteristics is of no greater metaphysical significance than this causal history featuring the actions of, say, antibiotic treatment or selective breeding. Thirdly, mental disorders can be natural kinds even if functionalism about the mind is correct. Even if Martian depression and human depression are physically very different, all cases of human depression may yet be physically similar. I conclude that there is thus no reason to rule out the possibility that some mental disorders might be natural kinds.

On investigation, it is plausible that some types of mental disorder are natural kinds, and that others are not. If mental disorders are natural kinds this is important because it will ground natural-history style explanations and predictions in psychiatry. Finally, we noted that saying that a mental disorder is a natural kind does not imply that people who suffer from it cannot be helped.

To finish, it is worth returning to our overall project of seeing how psychiatry is like other sciences. We can note that in so far as psychiatry employs natural-history style explanations and predictions it resembles the other sciences of natural history: field biology, geology and so on. Philosophical accounts of prediction and explanation that work for these sciences can be expected to work for psychiatry as well.

We can also expect that natural history within psychiatry may be shaped by social and financial pressures somewhat similar to those that have shaped natural history within other sciences. Recent work by some historians of science (Pickstone 2000; Jardine *et al.* 1996) suggests that natural-history style science has been far more important than one would guess from a cursory glance at typical texts in the history, sociology and philosophy of science. Observers of science have been seduced by the appeals of theory or, in more recent years, experiment, and it has been all too easy to forget that Big Science was once natural historical science. Still, while today experiments, such as those of CERN and the Human Genome Project, get the lion's share of funding, in the eighteenth and nineteenth centuries imperial powers invested in collections of plants, animals and rocks (such as those housed in the Natural History Museum in London). These collections enabled powerful nations to classify, and thus control, the resources and threats of their colonies. With museums and botanical gardens, useful plants, agricultural crops and the agents of human disease could all be studied and governed. Now, with empires dispersed, such collections have largely lost their allure (although they remain of some importance for both agriculture and industry).

This historical work on natural history shows that in other sciences natural history has been important because it enables one to control the world. In addition, it has been financed because such control can be exploited for monetary gain. I suggest that the case of psychiatry is no different. In classifying disorders we hope to gain control over them. In particular, one can hope that when drug treatments are found they will work for all patients who suffer from a particular kind of disorder. Here, as with the other natural history sciences, such hopes can be converted into money. A drug that works for all patients of a kind can potentially be sold to all patients of a kind. Plausibly, it is thus no accident that the massive expansion of interest in classification in psychiatry that has occurred since the 1970s coincides with the emergence of effective, and marketable, medications.[7] In some cases the link between the pharmaceutical industry and the promotion of natural-history style thinking in psychiatry is direct and explicit. Lakoff (2005) reports that in Argentina drug companies print and distribute Spanish-language editions of the DSM-IV. As one of his respondents tells him "In Argentina, the boom of the pharmaceutical industry in the last fifteen years has been notable, more or less coinciding with the beginning of the reading of DSM" (*ibid*.: 150). One can conjecture that, in the same way that zoology, botany and geology were once intimately connected with the needs of empire, psychiatric classification in the twenty-first century will be bound up with the needs of the pharmaceutical industry. The natural history sciences are important because classifying the world enables us to control it – and they are financed when there is money to be made from this control.

5. Explanations in psychiatry 2
Individual case histories

In this chapter we turn to a different and contrasting form of explanation that is also frequently found in psychiatry. We shall consider explanations provided by case histories that seek to make sense of a person's behaviour in terms of his or her psychological states. I want to explore how such case histories provide explanations, the circumstances under which they can fail and the extent to which the use of case histories in psychiatry suggests that psychiatry is like other sciences. To these ends, I shall explore how recent simulation accounts of folk-psychological understanding can help us understand how such case histories work.

5.1 The simulation account of folk-psychological understanding

Often we can predict the future behaviour of systems either by using theory or by using a simulation. To take a frequently used example, suppose we are building a bridge and want to know whether our design will withstand the winds in a particular valley. We might work this out in either of two ways: we might use a theory, and using the laws of physics do various calculations to see if the bridge is strong enough; or we might use a simulation, and predict the behaviour of the bridge by making a scale model and placing it in a wind tunnel. When we use a simulation to predict, we use a system that is analogous to the target system and reason that the two can be expected to behave similarly.

"Folk psychology" refers to the ways in which normal people (the "folk") predict and explain each other's mental states. Currently debate rages over the method that folk psychology employs. Simulationists think that we use a simulation-based method, about which more will be said later. Theory-theorists think we use a theory. They claim that we have a tacit understanding of laws that link various types of mental state, which we postulate as theoretical entities. Apart from the pure simulationists, and pure theory-theorists, many think we use both simulation and theory, and a minority think we use neither. There is no room here to review the debates between these distinct camps.[1] Instead, for the purposes of this chapter I shall merely assume that we at least sometimes gain understanding of others via simulation and consider how such an account can help us to understand how case histories work.

Simulationists claim that when we want to understand or predict others we use our own mental processes to simulate theirs. Suppose, for example, that I have arranged to meet a friend outside a railway station. I get there an hour late, the waiting room is closed, it is pouring with rain and I cannot see my friend. I need to predict where she has gone and what reception I may get when I find her. To solve these problems I imagine what I would do and feel in her situation: suppose it were me who has arrived to meet someone who has not shown up and is now getting wet. In such a situation, I would soon get quite annoyed. I conclude that she too is probably not very happy. After a while I would look for the nearest shelter. I conclude that she will have done likewise. I look around and see a nearby pub. And, when I go in, I find that my friend is there and that I am no longer very popular.

In the station case I merely had to imagine what I would think if I were in my friend's situation and I could conclude that she would think similarly. But in other cases we have to make allowances for the fact that the person we are trying to simulate is different from us. For example, I hate nuts, but I know that Sue likes them. I want to predict how Sue will act if she finds an unopened packet of nuts that is six months out of date down the back of her sofa. How do I go about doing this? Well, I can imagine that I do like nuts, and then imagine myself finding the packet down the back of the sofa. Or, I can imagine how I would act if I found a packet of something that I do like, such as jelly beans. Either way, I can conclude that Sue will be disappointed that the nuts are out of date, and rather shocked at the thought that she has not cleaned properly for six months.

Simulation-style accounts have been proposed by a number of philosophers over the past decade or so. The details of the accounts differ between writers. The best-known accounts can be thought of as ranging along a scale depending on the extent to which they are proposed on conceptual or empirical grounds. At one end of the scale Jane Heal (2003) presents an *a priori* argument for simulation, or co-cognition as she tends to call it. According to Heal one implication of our fundamental belief that others are rational is that we will think about what others think about in broadly the way that they do. Thus, if you are trying to find the post office, I can predict how you will act by thinking about what I would have reason to do in your circumstances. In that situation, any of us would have reason to look at a town map, or to ask a passer-by for directions. At the other end of the scale, Susan Hurley (2005) has presented an account that makes full use of the latest neuroscientific findings. Her account involves mirror neurons and a complex arrangement of sub-personal mental systems. Goldman's account is somewhere in the middle (2006: §2.2). His account makes some empirical claims about the structure of the mind, but without the neurological details involved in Hurley's account. Goldman thinks that there is a bit of our mind that we use to "run" pretend beliefs and desires in "off-line" simulations. Here we need not get drawn into the details of the various simulation accounts. The important thing for us is the idea that we might be able to predict and explain others' mental states by using our own mental processes to simulate theirs.

5.2 Simulation and case histories

My suggestion with regard to case histories is quite straightforward: it is that case histories work by providing us with the scaffolding to simulate another. This explains why case histories focus on all that is unique to the individual. I can suppose that most of another's mental states and ways of thinking will be the same as my own (they too will think that 2 + 2 = 4, that Paris is in France, that good food is nice, that being wet and cold is bad, and so on). As such, it is their peculiarities that I need to know about if I am to make the necessary corrections to my own ways of thinking to be able to mimic theirs. Along similar lines, the more detail provided by a case history the better it will tend to be. The more information I am given about another, the easier it will become for me to think as if I were them.

As an example of a case history that provides the scaffolding we need to simulate another, consider the case of Mary, presented by Robert Akeret (1995). One slight difficulty that I have here is that I think that the longer and more detailed a case history is the better it will tend to be. Here, however, there is no room to present full case histories, so we must make do with a case history sketch. Akeret's patient, Mary, had a Catholic upbringing. She had been brought up to believe that evil thoughts are approximately as bad as evil actions. As a child, on a number of occasions she had wished that bad things would happen to people, and they did. One day she became angry with her father and wished he were dead, and the next day he died. On the basis of this story we can easily imagine how we would feel if we had Mary's beliefs and were in her situation. It will come as no surprise to us that Mary suspects it is her fault that her father died, and that this leads to feelings of guilt and depression.

Thus, I suggest that case histories enable us to simulate another. We see that if we were in their situation we would think similarly. This gives us the beginnings of an explanation of their behaviour. Let us assume that we ourselves have fairly standard examples of human mental systems. Then, if we manage to simulate another, this gives us reason to think that human beings in general are likely to act or think as the subject does (when placed in the situation that they are in). In so far as we can simulate them, we can conclude that there is nothing special or abnormal about the subject. Any explanation of why they thought as they did in some particular circumstance will be an explanation of why any human being would think in that way in that circumstance.

This depends on the assumption that all human beings think in much the same way. But this in itself is a reasonable claim that can be argued for in at least two ways. As we have seen, Heal has argued that a fundamental part of our seeing ourselves and others as rational agents is that we assume that we will all think similarly. Roy Sorensen (1998) also argues for cognitive uniformity, but this time on evolutionary grounds. He thinks that there will be selective pressures that encourage cognitive uniformity; human beings who think alike will be better fitted to cooperate with others who think like them.

There is a tradition that has it that empathy is good only for generating hypotheses but not for testing them. Thus Ernst Nagel states that:

> The fact that the social scientist, unlike the student of inanimate nature, is able to project himself by sympathetic imagination into the phenomena he is attempting to understand, is pertinent to questions concerning the origins of his explanatory hypotheses but not to questions concerning their validity. (1961: 484–5)

By linking understanding another with simulating them we can see that Nagel is being too harsh. Suppose that in understanding another we simulate them. Whenever we can simulate one system with another we learn something about the behaviour that is simulated: we learn that the behaviour is standard for systems of that kind in that setting. This delimits the type of explanation that we should seek in explaining the system's behaviour: In so far as the target system can be simulated, the explanation of its behaviour must refer to features that are shared with the simulating system. Of course, we may still want an explanation of why it is that *any* of the systems behave as they do. When we simulate a system, this does not completely explain its behaviour, but it does at least tell us what kind of explanation we should look for.

5.3 What are the limits of simulation?

Many of the case histories to be found within psychiatry concern people who think in somewhat odd ways. Thus, in discussing how case histories are used in psychiatry we must consider whether there might be limits to the thoughts that we can simulate. Are there some people who think so strangely that we cannot simulate them?

Unfortunately, discussing the limits of simulation is somewhat problematic. How can we tell whether we are simulating? Is simulation under voluntary control? The answers to such questions will depend on the precise account of simulation that turns out to be correct. On some accounts, we simulate another by consciously deciding to run through thoughts like theirs. That is, we actively imagine ourselves in their situation. On such an account the process of simulation will presumably be open to introspection. We will thus know when we are simulating and whether we have got stuck. On other accounts, simulation may be involuntary and performed at a sub-personal level. If simulations are run by sub-personal systems, then introspection may not be able to inform us whether or not a simulation is still running.

In any case the best test of a successful simulation will be whether it enables one to predict successfully the actions or thoughts of another. It is a sad but commonplace truth that people frequently think they have understood things when they have not. As such we cannot just take the word of those who claim to understand at face value.

In discussing the limits of simulation I shall consider a range of cases where we might expect to run into difficulties. Simulation approaches to folk psychology are relatively new, and not much work has been done on the question of what the limits of simulation might be. Here I will survey some cases where others have suggested we might not be able to simulate, and offer a few possibilities of my own. The survey is intended to be suggestive rather than exhaustive.

5.3.1 Rationality

One might think that we can only simulate the rational (Heal 2003: 76). The plausibility of this claim depends on how "rational" is understood. The "rational" agent might be thought of as one who thinks in accord with the rules of formal logic, probability calculus and so on. Or, the rational agent might be one who thinks as normal human beings think.

I suggest that for us to simulate another they do not need to be rational in the sense of following the laws of logic; they just need to think in the same ways as we do.[2] To illustrate, consider the following case. Suppose that Jane is about to get into bed and finds a large spider on her pillow. I know she is averse to killing small creatures. What will she do? Given that spiders are harmless in the UK, it seems that the logically rational thing to do would be to pick up the spider with her hand and move it to the side of the bed. This is the easiest way of ensuring that the spider does not get squashed when Jane goes to sleep. But actually I predict that Jane will not do this. Instead, I predict that Jane will use some paper or a cup to move the spider outside her bedroom. Why? Because I predict that Jane, like myself and most other people, is somewhat averse to handling spiders. A low-level fear of spiders is not logically rational, but it is normal, and thus is automatically accommodated by my simulation. For me to simulate another they just need to think in the ways that I do.

5.3.2 Personal experience

For us to simulate others our mind has to work in a similar way to theirs. But do we also need to have had experiences similar to the ones they are going through? People frequently claim that one has to have gone through an experience oneself to really understand it. So, for example, medical students who have been hospitalized claim this improves their understanding of patients (Wilkes *et al.* 2002). Similarly, some within the mental health service user movement claim that users can better understand other users (e.g. Barnes & Shardlow 1996).

Many people think that personal experience improves understanding. I suspect they are right. However, although I have found plenty of people who are prepared to say that personal experience improves their ability to empathize, I have not been able to find any empirical evidence that indicates the extent to which this commonly held belief is actually true.

Even if we suppose that those who have gone through an experience themselves are more sympathetic, there may be different reasons why this is the case. It might be that those with personal experience are better able to simulate the thoughts of someone who is now going through a similar experience. So, for example, maybe a midwife who has had children herself can better simulate the thoughts of a woman in labour. On the other hand, the difference might be due to the person simply remembering that the experience was unpleasant and thus being more sympathetic. That is, the midwife might no longer be able to experience anything like the pains of childbirth but just remembers that it was horrible. Further empirical work would be required to determine whether it is generally true that personal experience enhances our ability to sympathise with others, and whether any such effects operate via an increased ability to simulate or via non-simulation-based memory.

5.3.3 Biological and chemical differences

It might be the case that we cannot simulate some minds because biological or chemical differences result in them working differently from our own. Such thoughts have inspired a minor tradition of psychiatrists taking mind-altering drugs in the hope that this will enable them to better understand their psychotic patients. Most such work was conducted in the 1950s and 1960s and involved psychiatrists taking LSD or mescaline in the hope of gaining insight into schizophrenic thought processes.

Fairly typical in this tradition is a 1956 study by John Macdonald and James Galvin called "Experimental Psychotic States" published in the *American Journal of Psychiatry*. A pharmaceutical company had given Macdonald and Galvin a large quantity of LSD. They gave much of it to their patients, but took some themselves. They considered that while on LSD "the psychiatrist may experience hallucinations, illusions, depersonalization, and other symptoms that he sees in his patients" (1956: 973).

There are a number of problems that one might note with such studies. Most obviously, one might doubt the extent to which LSD-induced mental processes can be expected to resemble schizophrenic mental processes. Plausibly different types of hallucinogenic drugs produce different types of experience, and the hallucinations produced in schizophrenia might be expected to differ yet again.

Let us place such concerns to one side, however, and ask whether if a drug did alter the mental processes of the psychiatrist such that they became similar to those of a psychotic patient, this would enable the psychiatrist to simulate the patient more easily. We can only simulate another to the extent that our mental processes are similar. Thus, to the extent that the drugs make the psychiatrist's mind like that of a psychotic patient the psychiatrist can expect to be able to simulate the psychotic. Here a problem emerges, however. While on the drugs many experimenters found that they lost interest in their research project. While in the state they need to be in if they are to simulate (i.e. on the drugs), they simply did not feel motivated to think about schizophrenic thought processes, or to describe their own experiences. In the MacDonald and Galvin study: "one of the writers found the phantasy world so entertaining that he became impatient when asked to describe it. The experience was too satisfying and the time too precious to be spent in describing this state of ecstasy" (1956: 972).

Psychiatrists on drugs are not interested in understanding psychotic thought patterns, but what about after the drug experiences? Could the psychiatrist who has experienced LSD-induced hallucinations simulate a psychotic patient when he is no longer on the drugs? Some psychiatrists have claimed that their drug induced experiences have enhanced their post-drug understanding of patients. John Kafka and Kenneth Gaarder (1964) gave psychiatrists LSD the day before they practised psychotherapy. Some of the psychiatrists felt that their drug experiences gave them a better understanding of behaviour that they had previously found peculiar. In particular, one patient would repeatedly ask her psychiatrist to come into her room so she could "explain things", but would then fall silent. Her psychiatrist reported that: "His LSD experience of the richness of the physiognomy of objects made this behaviour seem less bizarre since he could assume that she was silently asking him to share this richness" (1964: 240). However, although the psychiatrist considered his understanding to have been enhanced, there are reasons to be doubtful. There might be many different reasons why the patient acted as she did, and the therapist's claim that she was awestruck by the richness of her visual experiences is just a guess. Overall, I am sceptical of the idea that those who have taken drugs will be able to afterwards simulate what it is like to be on drugs. When someone has taken drugs their mind works in particular ways because of the chemical changes brought about by the drugs. These chemical changes are not available to consciousness, and so it would not be possible to reproduce them consciously when one wants to run a simulation at a later time (I guess this would be why it is not possible to get drunk-feelings by just thinking about drinking alcohol). This being said, although I do not think that LSD experiences will enable psychiatrists to better simulate psychotic patients, drug experiences may enable one to learn some things that will help one to be more sympathetic to psychotic patients. For example, an LSD experience might enable one to learn that hallucinations can be very frightening, and learning this might change how a psychiatrist interacts with patients.

5.3.4 Trauma

There may be some mental states that we have problems simulating because the situation of the subject is too horrific. Consider this vignette, which opens John Wilson and Rhiannon Thomas's *Empathy in the Treatment of Trauma and PTSD*:

> I was given another choice: I rape my daughter or the guard does. I tried to reason with them, telling them that she was an innocent child ... They laughed and repeated the two choices. I looked at my daughter hoping that she would tell me what to do – our eyes met and I knew that I could not save her from those wretched men. I lowered my eyes in shame to keep from seeing my daughter abused. One guard held my face up, forcing me to watch this horrible scene. I watched, motionless, as she was raped before me and her little brother. When they were through, they forced me to do what they had done to her. My own daughter, my son forced to watch it all. How could anyone do that? What kind of men are they? What kind of father am I?
>
> (Wilson & Thomas 2004: 3, citing Ortiz 2001: 18)

Some therapists claim that they can empathize with people who have undergone such events. I do not think I can. The problems are twofold. On the one hand the events described are far beyond the realms of my experience. I have never seen anyone raped, and I do not have any children. The other problem is that seeking to simulate terrible thoughts is disturbing. As such, it is very hard to force oneself to do it. The problem is that one tends to find oneself avoiding attempting the simulation. Thus, Wilson and Thomas found that many of the therapists they spoke to encountered difficulty in empathizing with trauma patients: therapists would find themselves thinking of other things, or falling asleep, to avoid having to pay attention. Somewhat similarly, Regehr *et al.* (2002) found that ambulance paramedics developed a whole range of techniques that enabled them to avoid empathizing with the victims of tragedy. The paramedics picked up bodies but avoided talking to the relatives of the dead, or they avoided empathizing with victims by concentrating on the technical details of what they needed to do next. When those who work with trauma victims do empathize with them, they frequently find this extremely upsetting. Those who empathize with trauma victims can find that they themselves experience intrusive imagery, nightmares and so on (*ibid.*). The problems that are faced by those who empathize with the victims of trauma also mean that it is hard for an individual to gain much experience in such work; rather than getting better at simulating the thoughts of the traumatized, the risk is that the person who works too long with trauma victims instead just becomes hardened or traumatized themselves.

It is worth noting that those who have experienced traumatic events themselves can also be expected to have problems simulating the thoughts of those going through similar events. Commonly, those who have undergone traumatic events have problems when they encounter stimuli that remind them of their trauma. Those who have been traumatized by war can end up panicking when they hear fireworks, for example. When a person who has been traumatized seeks to simulate the thoughts of someone in a similar situation it is likely that the affect generated will knock their thoughts off kilter. They will stop simulating and get caught up with their own unpleasant emotions.[3]

5.3.5 A predicted differential ability to simulate odd mental states

Many simulationists have emphasized that our ability to simulate is linked to our ability to think about what we ourselves would do in hypothetical situations.[4] Their thought is that it is useful for us to be able to plan: to think about what we will do if such and such turns out to the case. A side effect of our ability to do this is that we can also predict how others will behave. We just think about what we would do if we were in their situation.

If this is right, it suggests that we might find simulating some odd mental states easier than others. Our own mental states differ in their vulnerability to revision. We regularly have to change many of our beliefs as we discover new and surprising things. Beliefs such as "Milton Keynes is a boring place to live", "My friend John likes me" and "Runner beans are easy to grow" are highly revisable. I can imagine many scenarios in which I would be forced to change my mind on these matters. As such, I suggest, it is fairly easy to simulate someone who disagrees with me on such claims. In contrast, we rarely change our basic desires (that is, things that we desire for their own sake, such as food or sex). Some people's sexual interests revolve around rubber gloves or dead bodies, but I cannot imagine a scenario in which my sexual desires switched to such things, and have problems simulating such people. Along similar lines, certain "core beliefs" may be highly resistant to revision. I cannot imagine revising my belief that there are external objects, or that I am alive. Once again, trying to simulate someone without such beliefs seems difficult, if not impossible. Plausibly we can only simulate another if their mental states are ones that we ourselves might have had if the circumstances had been different, or that at least is my suggestion. Now for some examples to make it seem plausible.

An easy simulation: a case with different "peripheral" beliefs

The Maniac, first published anonymously in 1909, seeks to provide an account of madness from "the maniac's point of view". During her spell of mania, the maniac suffers from many delusions. At one point she comes out in severe acne (brought on, she thinks, by the medication she is being given), and starts to think that each spot is a "fat, white maggot, eating her alive" (Thelmar [1909] 1932: 188–9). It is, I suggest, quite easy to simulate someone who thinks that their spots contain maggots. Spots do look a bit maggoty, and we all know that there actually are some bugs that burrow inside the skin. It is easy to imagine situations in which we ourselves come to believe that there are insects inside us. And, it is easy to imagine the kinds of thoughts that would follow from thinking oneself maggot-infested. One can imagine alternately scratching the spots to try to get the maggots out, and then being too repulsed to touch them, for example (indeed writing this my skin is crawling already).

I can imagine thinking myself maggot-infested and can simulate someone who thinks this. Similarly, it is comparatively easy to simulate the thoughts of someone who comes to believe that their friends all hate them, or that they can write brilliant poetry, for example. Here again, we can imagine many scenarios in which we ourselves might come to hold such beliefs.

A hard simulation: a case with different basic desires

The title case of Robert Akeret's *The Man Who Loved a Polar Bear* (1995) concerns Charles, a man who falls in love, in a sexual way, with a polar bear called Zero. After his amorous advances lead to injury, Charles goes to consult Akeret. At one stage Akeret goes with Charles to meet Zero. Looking at the bear, Akeret finds it hard to empathize with Charles. He writes: "At that moment I tried with all of my imagination to empathize with Charles, to feel what it would be like to love this bear as a man loves a woman. To lust after her. I confess that I could not do that" (1995: 82).

Simulating odd desires can clearly be harder than simulating odd peripheral beliefs. This being said, we can simulate at least some of those whose desires differ from our own. In some cases another's desires can be seen as analogous to my own. So, suppose I do not find my friend's boyfriend at all attractive. Still I can simulate what her thoughts would be if she walked in to find him in bed with another woman. I can imagine how I would feel in such a situation if it involved my partner and conclude that her feelings will be similar.

Still, I suggest, this process has limits. I do not think I can simulate how Charles would feel if he turned up at Zero's cage to find her snuggled up to a he-bear. On the one hand, if Charles is in love with Zero one can expect him to feel jealous. On the other hand, jealousy normally involves the thought that one could fill the place taken by another, whereas in the case of Zero and her bear-lover the reasons for Zero's preferences would be fairly clear. All in all, I do not think I can simulate how Charles would feel in such a situation. I have no idea how his thoughts would go.

Maybe my problems with simulating Charles are merely down to a lack of imagination on my part, but at any rate, there seem to be clear-cut limits to the desires that we can simulate. Plausibly we cannot simulate desires in cases where we desire nothing analogous. So prior to becoming interested in sex, the idea of sex seems disgusting. Similarly, it is hard to simulate someone who feels compelled to tear their hair out if we lack such desires ourselves, for example.

An even harder simulation

Consider a patient who says the following:

> I have not eaten for months / or gone to the toilet / all the organs within me have rotten / the food can't pass through, everything has been coagulated / the Lonarid (paracetamol) that I took, have stuffed my bowel, this is unfortunately my punishment / I am tired, I haven't slept for years / I have no blood / I have no heart, it doesn't beat anymore. I was deceived at the ECG department while they knew that my heart doesn't beat anymore / you are deceiving me when you take my blood pressure, because I'm not alive anymore, I'm a dead-plant.
>
> (Vaxevanis and Vidalis 2005: 42)

This quote is from a patient suffering from Cotard's delusion. Importantly for the example, people with Cotard's believe they are dead in the sense of non-being, rather than thinking that they have died and gone to heaven or hell. If we try to simulate the thoughts of such a person I suggest we just get stuck. I cannot think of any situation in which I would come to believe that I am dead. Furthermore, if by chance I did come to believe I was dead, I do not know what other thoughts would follow. If you believe you are dead do you look for a doctor, or an undertaker? Suppose you go and see the undertaker and try to arrange your own funeral, how do you account for the fact that you can talk with the undertaker, walk around and get hungry?

The basic problem with trying to simulate such thoughts is that we cannot think of any circumstances in which we would come to share such thoughts ourselves. Along somewhat similar lines, in his discussion of Cotard's delusion, John Campbell (2001) suggests that such patients may be incomprehensible to the rest of us because they hold different "framework propositions". In *On Certainty* (1969), Wittgenstein talks about the epistemic status of propositions such as "The world has existed for quite a long time" and "There are a lot of objects in the world". Unlike most propositions, such "framework propositions" are not open to doubt. Rather, other propositions are judged against them. As Campbell puts it: "it is only when we have the framework propositions in play, assumed to be correct, that it makes any sense to try to establish whether any proposition agrees with reality or not; we need the framework propositions in order to have any methods for testing at all" (2001: 96). Campbell's suggestion is that patients with Cotard's delusion take "I am dead" as a framework proposition. This is why the proposition is treated as something that is taken for granted and that is immune to revision. In Campbell's account, it is because our framework propositions differ from the patient's that we cannot imagine thinking like them.

To sum up, it is plausible that we can only simulate another when we ourselves could come to have their thoughts, or at least thoughts analogous to their thoughts. Simulating those whose peripheral beliefs differ from our own is thus easier than simulating those with very different basic desires or different core beliefs.

5.3.6 Unconscious mental states

So far the simulations we have considered involve simulating conscious beliefs and desires, but what of unconscious beliefs and desires? I suggest that the traditional case histories of psychoanalysis do not work purely via simulation. At key points we cannot track unconscious thoughts via simulation, but have to appeal to other resources (e.g. psychoanalytic theory). I shall try to make this claim plausible by considering an example drawn from one of Freud's cases: the "Rat man". Freud reports the following:

> One day while he was away on his summer holidays the idea suddenly occurred to him that he was too fat [German "dick"] and that he must *make himself slimmer*. So he began getting up from table before the pudding came round and tearing along the road without a hat in the blazing heat of an August sun. Then he would dash up a mountain at the double, till, dripping with perspiration, he was forced to come to a stop .... Our patient could think of no explanation of this senseless obsessional behaviour until it suddenly occurred to him that at that

> time his lady had also been stopping at the same resort; but she had been in the company of an English cousin, who was very attentive to her and of whom the patient had been very jealous. This cousin's name was Richard, and according to the usual practice in England, he was known as *Dick*. Our patient, then, had wanted to kill this Dick; he had been far more jealous of him and enraged with him than he could admit to himself, and that was why he had imposed on himself this course of slimming by way of a punishment. (Freud [1909] 1991: 69)

Here I suggest we cannot follow the thoughts of the patient simply via simulation. If I suppose that I am jealous of someone called Richard, and allow my mind to simulate what follows, I do not conclude that going running will be a good idea. From the simulation I would probably just conclude that I shall be a bit upset and might be unkind to Richard. Instead of working via simulation, Freud's explanation requires psychoanalytic theory. One needs to accept certain theoretical claims, such as that thoughts can be repressed and manifest themselves in disguised ways, before the case history makes sense. As Freud himself puts it, in this case the link between the cause and the symptoms "succeeded in concealing itself behind one of those purely external associations which are so obnoxious to our consciousness" (*ibid.*: 68). As the unconscious links thoughts in different ways than does the conscious, we cannot simulate unconscious thoughts in the same way that we can simulate conscious ones.

To summarize, I suggest that on a simulation-based account we may expect to have problems simulating certain others. In particular, we may have problems simulating those whose minds work differently from our own, people who have undergone traumatic experiences, people whose core beliefs or basic desires differ from our own and unconscious mental states.

5.4 Returning to tradition: this account of case histories compared with others

Traditionally, those who discuss case histories appeal to the importance of "narrative understanding", "empathy" or "*Verstehen*". It is worth noting that the simulation account offered here is compatible with these traditions. I can say that *Verstehen*, empathy or narrative understanding work via simulation.[5] Here we shall briefly consider the claims of Karl Jaspers, the writer most discussed in psychiatry in relation to case histories, to show how my account can be used to flesh out traditional claims about the operation of case histories.

As is well known, Jaspers draws an important distinction between explanation and understanding. Explanations are characteristically found in the physical sciences: they explain why something happens by appealing to laws. Understanding is different. According to Jaspers we understand how psychic reactions emerge out of one another in a way that is self-evident and basic. He writes:

> When Nietzsche shows how an awareness of one's weakness, wretchedness and suffering gives rise to moral demands and religions of redemption, because in this roundabout way the psyche can gratify its will to power in spite of its weakness, we experience the force of his argument and are convinced. It strikes us as something self-evident which cannot be broken down any further. ([1923] 1963: 303)

Jaspers does not say very much about how understanding is supposed to work,[6] although he does mention that a distinction should be drawn between rational understanding and true empathy. As he puts it:

> thoughts may be understandable because they emerge from each other according to the rules of logic and here the connections are understood rationally (we understand what is said). But where we understand how certain thoughts rise from moods, wishes or fears, we are understanding the connections in the true psychological sense, that is by empathy (we understand the speaker). (*Ibid.*: 304)

Thus, in essence, Jaspers claims that true empathy is a basic form of understanding about which nothing much can be said, which is not very helpful. With the account sketched in this chapter, however, we can flesh out Jaspers's claims. We can say that simulation allows us to predict how thoughts rise from wishes and fears. When it comes to Jaspers's category of rational understanding, I suggest that sometimes we simulate how beliefs are logically related and sometimes we might use other means. If I assume that you are quite good at logic, then I might predict the conclusions that you will draw from various beliefs using the rules of logic, or I might simulate you by pretending that I share your beliefs and seeing what conclusions I draw. I suggest that the account of case histories proposed here is not in conflict with traditional claims about the importance of empathy, *Verstehen*, narrative understanding and so on, but can be understood as an account of how such forms of understanding might operate.

5.5 Ethics and case histories

A long tradition in psychiatry has it that a case-history-based approach is in some way more ethical than a theory-based approach. One benefit of a simulation-based approach to case histories is that it gives an account of the ethical superiorities of case histories. Simulating another is very closely linked to empathizing with another.[7] When we simulate other peoples' mental states this forces us to consider them as people with beliefs, hopes and fears, and to try to see the world from their point of view. This is important because once we have taken on board that another person has interests that differ from our own it is harder to then act in ways that ignore these interests. Thus, those who listen to the personal histories of psychiatric patients are perhaps less likely to act in ways that deny the humanity of such patients. One point that fits in with the suggestion that case histories promote empathy is that reading case histories tends to have a different effect on people than reading theory-based psychiatric explanations. While theory-based explanations provoke curiosity, case histories can make readers cry (Roberts 2000). A simulation-based approach to case histories explains why it is that reading case histories would be phenomenologically distinct from reading theories.

5.6 Conclusion

To summarize, in this chapter I have suggested that a simulation-based approach can help us make sense of case histories. On my account, case histories work by providing us with the scaffolding necessary to simulate the thoughts of another. In so far as we can simulate another we can conclude that they think in ways that are normal for human beings under the circumstances. Plausibly, there are limits to what we can simulate. We may have problems simulating: (i) people whose minds work differently from our own; (ii) people who have undergone traumatic experiences; (iii) people whose core beliefs or basic desires differ from our own; and (iv) unconscious mental states. I suggest that the simulation account of case histories proposed here is compatible with traditional accounts of case histories that talk of empathy, *Verstehen* or narrative understanding. Finally, we can note that simulating another is linked to empathizing with them. This explains why a case-history-based approach may have ethical advantages.

To return to the question of the extent to which psychiatry is like or unlike other disciplines, we can conclude that in so far as psychiatry makes use of case histories that explain by citing a person's intentional mental states, the explanations provided by psychiatry can be considered alongside those provided by areas of history and anthropology that use similar types of explanation. More broadly, to the extent that such case studies can be regarded as a species of simulation-based explanation, psychiatry can be considered alongside all sciences that use simulations to explain.

In this chapter and Chapter 4 we have looked at two forms of explanation that are frequently found in psychiatry but are less common in other sciences, namely natural-history style explanations and individual case histories. It may be worth restating that these are, of course, not the only types of explanation found in psychiatry. Other types of explanation are also found (e.g. explanation based on non-strict laws, cognitive modelling and evolutionary hypotheses). Here we have focused on natural-history-based explanations and case histories simply because these types of explanation have been little explored by philosophers of science to date.

6. Relations between theories 1
When paradigms meet

Characteristically, within psychiatry there is agreement over little. Instead there tend to be many competing schools and theories. Chapters 6 and 7 examine how distinct schools of thought relate to each other. This chapter looks at what happens when distinct paradigms meet. In particular it considers the extent to which communication between paradigms is possible. Chapter 7 looks at reductionism, and considers when one theory can be reduced to another.

Famously, Kuhn (1970) claimed that scientists normally work within paradigms, and that communication across paradigms is problematic. We shall shortly look at Kuhn's position in greater detail, but in very brief outline Kuhn holds that scientists working in different paradigms see the world in different ways, their theoretical terms have different meanings, and they have different assumptions and values. As a consequence, when they talk to each other, they talk past each other.

Psychiatry is an especially interesting case in considering Kuhn's arguments. In most scientific sub-disciplines all those working on a problem at a time work within the same paradigm. In psychiatry, however, competing groups of scientists adhere to radically different theoretical frameworks. What is more, as many mental health practitioners work in multidisciplinary teams, most mental health professionals have to try to communicate with others who do not share their theoretical commitments on a daily basis.

In this chapter I shall examine whether Kuhn's picture of science can accommodate disciplines like psychiatry. I shall assess the extent to which different mental health practitioners can be said to work within different paradigms, and the extent to which they have problems communicating with each other. I argue that Kuhn's more radical claims cannot be substantiated. Luckily, communication across different paradigms is not as problematic as he suggests. Readers already familiar with Kuhn's work can skip the first two sections.

6.1 Kuhn on paradigms and normal science

Kuhn's 1962 work *The Structure of Scientific Revolutions* is one of the most influential books written in the philosophy of science in the twentieth century. Kuhn was trained as a physicist. He was taught that science is progressive, that good scientists are constantly questioning their theories, and that decisions between scientific theories are normally made on rational grounds. However, studying the history of science led him to conclude that fairly much everything he had been told about science was false. Accordingly, in *The Structure of Scientific Revolutions*, Kuhn presents us with a radically different picture of the scientific enterprise. Kuhn's favourite examples are drawn from physics and chemistry. In setting out his views I shall stick to examples from these sciences. Then, in §6.3, I go on to examine whether and how his views apply to psychiatry.

According to Kuhn, the history of science consists mainly of long periods of "normal science". During periods of normal science everyone working in a sub-discipline structures their work according to some particular "paradigm". Scientists working under a particular paradigm agree on the framework in which they conduct their research. Scientists who share a paradigm will agree on the following:

- the types of questions that are worth asking;
- the types of method to be used in answering them, that is, they agree on what instruments to use, on appropriate statistical techniques and so on;
- metaphysical constraints on answers – for example, in a particular paradigm action-at-a-distance may not be allowed;
- what counts as good work – they will broadly agree on which papers count as excellent within their field.

In addition, they have access to a similar set of skills. They will be able to perform similar types of research.

During periods of normal science the whole of a sub-discipline takes it for granted that their paradigm is broadly correct. Scientists working within the paradigm of Newtonian mechanics, for example, assume that Newton's laws are right. The fundamental theoretical claims of the paradigm are not questioned. Assuming the correctness of the paradigm is generally a good strategy. It means that scientists do not have to spend time figuring out the answers to fundamental questions for themselves. Instead of worrying about basic theoretical questions, scientists working within the paradigm fiddle around solving "puzzles": they might show how the paradigm can be extended to a new area, and, for example, work on applying the laws of mechanics to the flow of liquids; or they might refine the equipment needed to measure theoretically important results, and aim, for example, to measure G, the gravitational constant, with ever greater accuracy. As scientists concentrate on specialized areas, and generally pick the problems that look easiest, during normal science many puzzles are solved.

When scientists fail to solve a puzzle this is generally taken to show that more ingenuity is required rather than that there is any fundamental problem with the paradigm. For the most part this assumption is justified: solutions to most puzzles are eventually found. However, sometimes things will not turn out as the paradigm says they should. Maybe a scientist will observe something that the paradigm cannot account for. Maybe some problem will keep resisting solution. Such difficulties are called anomalies.

Usually, when scientists come across anomalies they ignore them. Normal science rewards scientists for solving puzzles, not for pointing out problems. Scientists have no motivation to draw attention to anomalies because their peers will probably assume that if an experiment went wrong then this is simply because the scientist is incompetent. In some cases, however, continuing to ignore an anomaly ceases to be a viable response. Maybe the anomaly is simply too striking to ignore; maybe there are strong external pressures to sort out the problem, for example, because a solution is needed for social or economic reasons.

If anomalies keep building up, then eventually a scientific community will come to see itself as being in a state of crisis. The scientists will begin to lose faith in their paradigm. As problems continue to resist solution scientists will start bending the rules under which they had been working in ever more desperate attempts to find a solution. During periods of crisis, scientists start to ask questions that they do not ask during periods of normal science. They start to engage in increasingly metaphysical speculation. Some will start to wonder whether the view of reality implicit in their paradigm might be wrong.

Eventually, a scientist may come up with a new paradigm, that is, with a new way of looking at the domain in question. If the new paradigm looks promising enough it may win over converts from the old paradigm. If enough scientists begin working under the new paradigm a new period of normal science begins. Thus, for Kuhn, the history of science can be seen to consist of long periods of normal science, punctuated by occasional crises and revolutions.

6.2 Kuhn on incommensurability

One of Kuhn's most controversial claims is that paradigms are "incommensurable". This means that there is no objective, external standard by which the paradigms can be compared. There is no fair way of deciding which of two paradigms is the better.

Kuhn thinks paradigms are incommensurable for three main reasons:

- perception is paradigm dependent;
- meaning is paradigm dependent; and
- the importance attributed to different factors is paradigm dependent.

6.2.1 Perception is paradigm dependent

Kuhn claims that what scientists observe depends on their theoretical beliefs. Scientists working under different paradigms have different theoretical beliefs and so see different things. In support of this claim, Kuhn cites a number of psychological experiments, most memorably a famous experiment by Jerome Bruner and Leo Postman (Kuhn 1970: 62–3). In the experiment, subjects were shown playing cards very quickly and asked to identify them. Some of the cards were anomalous, for example, a black six of hearts. Bruner and Postman found that subjects tended to see the anomalous cards as being completely normal. Thus they might report a black six of hearts as being a six of spades, for example. The subjects saw what they expected to see.

Like the subjects in the experiment, Kuhn claims that scientists have a tendency to see what they anticipate they will see. As an example, Kuhn discusses how Aristotelian astronomers failed to observe comets. According to Aristotelian views of the universe the heavens should be immutable, that is they should not change. Heavenly bodies are neither created nor destroyed and continue in circular orbits forever. According to this theory comets should not exist and so the astronomers failed to notice them. In contrast, Kuhn claims, Chinese astronomers had no belief that the heavens were constant, and they spotted numerous comets.

Because scientists working under different paradigms see different things, the world looks different to the different scientists.

6.2.2 Meaning is paradigm dependent

Scientists working under different paradigms may use the same words. They may both talk of "atoms", for example. However, Kuhn claims that when a word such as "atom" is used by scientists working in different paradigms it may mean different things. Kuhn thinks that the meaning of theoretical terms can vary with paradigm because he thinks that the meaning of theoretical terms is given by their place in a theory. To see why such a view is plausible, consider how one learns the meaning of a theoretical term such as "atom". When someone is being taught what atoms are they will be told, for example, that molecules are made up of atoms and atoms are made up of electrons, neutrons and protons. It is only possible to learn what "atom" means if one also learns a whole network of concepts that go with it. The meaning of "atom" is given by its place in the theory. As such, when scientists with different theories about atoms use a term such as "atom" they mean different things.

To see how this can lead to problems with communication across paradigms consider what would happen if (time travel permitting) an ancient Greek were to talk about atoms with a modern scientist. As is well known, some ancient Greeks believed that matter is made up of atoms. For them, atoms were the smallest pieces of matter; they could not be divided any further. Contemporary scientists also believe in atoms. However, they think that atoms are made up of more fundamental particles: electrons, protons and neutrons. Now imagine an ancient Greek and a contemporary scientist having an argument over whether or not atoms can be divided. The ancient Greek will say that they are indivisible. For him "atom" means "thing that can be divided no further". The contemporary scientist will say they can be divided. However, neither scientist will be able to persuade the other, as the two will be talking at cross-purposes.

6.2.3 The importance attributed to different factors is paradigm dependent

Paradigms can differ from each other in a wide variety of different ways, for example:

- the extent to which they can account for empirical observations;
- their scope;
- their mathematical elegance;
- the numbers of different types of entity they posit; and
- their technological promise.

It is most likely that one paradigm will score better than another on some of these grounds, but not on others. How, then, is the importance of each of the above criteria to be weighted? Kuhn claims that the importance given to simplicity, say, or empirical accuracy will depend on a scientist's paradigm. Once again, this means that there is no external standard against which the paradigms can be compared.

To sum up, Kuhn thinks that scientists working in different paradigms will see the world differently, their theoretical terms have different meanings and they value theories with different features. As a consequence, paradigms are incommensurable. There is no objective, external standard that can be used to adjudicate between paradigms.

If paradigms cannot be fairly compared, one paradigm cannot be proved better than another. Why, then, do scientists switch from one paradigm to another? Kuhn's answer is that they switch for their own idiosyncratic reasons:

maybe the new paradigm solves some problem that seemed to them to be especially pressing; maybe proponents of the new paradigm have secured funding; maybe the paradigm appeals to them on aesthetic or metaphysical grounds. For whatever reasons, they switch sides. If enough scientists convert to the new paradigm, then it will take over from the old paradigm.

Scientists must either work under one paradigm or under another. Paradigms cannot be changed a little bit at a time. So, when scientists convert to the new paradigm they do so wholesale. Kuhn likens the switch from one paradigm to another to a religious conversion. If someone has been an atheist and then starts to believe in God then their whole life changes; everything about the world begins to look different to them. Similarly, for scientists who switch paradigms, the domain in which they work appears completely new: new questions seem interesting, new methods appropriate, new results relevant.

Inevitably, some scientists will refuse to switch to the new paradigm. If the new paradigm is successful in winning enough converts, then those who cling to the old paradigm will become marginalized. They will not be able to get papers published, and as they die, the old paradigm will die with them.

6.3 Paradigms in psychiatry

Most of Kuhn's examples are taken from physics or chemistry. Based on his studies of these sciences, Kuhn concluded that ordinarily during normal science, the whole of a scientific sub-discipline works under one paradigm.[1] Kuhn expects this to be the case because he thinks that unless the community is prepared to take much for granted then it will spend so long arguing over fundamentals that it will make little progress.

In this section I argue that the "psych-sciences" – that is, psychiatry, psychology, psychoanalysis and allied disciplines – differ from many other sciences in that they are multi-paradigm sciences. Competing schools of thought coexist. To focus in on two particular approaches, we shall consider biologically oriented psychiatry and psychoanalysis. In her book, *Of Two Minds: The Growing Disorder in American Psychiatry*, anthropologist of science Tanya Luhrmann explores the state of US psychiatry in the early 1990s. She finds major splits between biologically oriented psychiatry and psychoanalysis. According to Luhrmann:

> Psychiatrists are taught to listen to people in particular ways: they listen for signals most of us cannot hear, and they look for patterns most of us cannot see. Their two primary tasks, however – diagnosis and psychopharmacology, on the one hand, and psychodynamic psychotherapy, on the other – teach them to listen and look in different ways. (2000: 22)

Luhrmann describes how young biologically oriented psychiatrists learn to spot disorders immediately. They see one patient as suffering from schizophrenia, and another as suffering from anxiety, in "the way plane spotters can spot Boeing 747s, the way bird-watchers can spot great snowy owls" (*ibid.*: 35). In contrast, psychoanalysts "listen for the stories that emerge from the way people talk about other people, the way they experience those people, the way they experience the therapist, and the way they experience themselves" (*ibid.*: 57).

The two groups ask different types of questions and evaluate treatments differently. Biologically oriented psychiatrists ask questions about neurotransmitters and the genetic components of disorder. They believe that the right way to assess new treatments is via double-blind clinical trials. In contrast, psychoanalysts are interested in the stories behind their patients' lives. They value case studies over experiments.

Biologically oriented psychiatry and psychoanalysis clearly constitute distinct Kuhnian paradigms. Furthermore, these are not the only paradigms in the psych-sciences. Social, behaviourist and cognitive approaches also constitute distinct paradigms. Kuhn thought there would only be one paradigm in a sub-discipline at a time, but within the psych-sciences, I claim, there are multiple competing paradigms. In his book *The Philosophical Defence of Psychiatry* (1991), Reznek disagrees. He argues that the different schools in psychiatry do not constitute distinct paradigms because they all agree that abnormal processes lead to suffering and disability. The mistake Reznek makes here is to think that such limited theoretical consistency is sufficient for researchers to share a paradigm. As we have seen, those who share a paradigm do not just agree on a few claims; they also see the world in a similar way, they think that the same questions are important, and conduct the same style of research. Once these factors are taken into account it becomes clear that the different schools within psychiatry constitute distinct paradigms.

I suggest that the reason that it is possible to have multiple paradigms in mental health is that there is an abundance of investigators in these areas. Kuhn looked mainly at pre-twentieth-century physics and chemistry. Based on his cases, he estimated that the size of the community that shares a paradigm might be fewer than twenty-five scientists (1970: 181). When only a small number of scientists work in a sub-discipline, the whole community has to work under one paradigm for progress to be made. If the community does not share a paradigm they will waste too much time arguing about fundamentals for progress to be possible. Currently, however, the sheer numbers of mental health professionals who conduct research means that multiple paradigms can be supported. Numbers are such that each school can support its own journals and conferences and carry on in semi-independence from other schools. When addressing colleagues using a particular paradigm, researchers in the psych-sciences can assume a shared background of assumptions and get on with the puzzle-solving that is characteristic of Kuhnian normal science.

At this point some might suggest that the psych-sciences should not be considered multi-paradigm sciences but are rather simply pre-sciences. A discipline is pre-scientific when it is still searching for its first paradigm. Kuhn himself says that the existence of competing schools is indicative of a pre-science. During pre-science there is no overall consensus as to the direction research should take, and as such debates over fundamentals are commonplace. According to Kuhn, it is only once one school meets with success and wins over enough supporters that normal science can begin. Maybe the existence of competing schools within the psych-sciences indicates that these are pre-sciences that are still in search of their first paradigm?

I suggest that this possibility should be rejected. In pre-science each thinker has to start by arguing for the foundations of his or her position. This is not necessary for researchers in the psych-sciences. Consider, for example, a typical paper that discusses possible susceptibility genes in schizophrenia. The authors of such papers do not spend time arguing for the reality of schizophrenia, or for the plausibility that there might be a genetic element (although such points are contested by other scientists in the field); rather, they assume that their audience will be familiar with their working assumptions and are just able to get on with discussing the details of their study. Such practices are characteristic of normal science.

I conclude that the psych-sciences offer genuine examples of sciences where the existence of multiple paradigms within a sub-discipline is the norm. Once this is accepted interesting questions emerge. Kuhn claims that scientists working within different paradigms will have problems communicating. In most sciences this claim is hard to test as revolutions are rare and last only for a comparatively short time. However, multi-paradigm sub-disciplines are the norm in the psych-sciences. Are there problems with communication, as Kuhn would lead us to expect? Or, if practitioners working within different paradigms can communicate, how do they achieve this? The remainder of this chapter will be devoted to examining whether and how communication occurs between the different paradigms in the psych-sciences.

6.4 An extra problem Kuhn does not discuss: inter-professional rivalry

Much mental health care is delivered by multidisciplinary teams. Such a team might consist of a psychiatrist, a psychologist, two social workers and three community psychiatric nurses, for example. The members of such teams think within different paradigms. Tony Colombo *et al.* (2003) studied how the members of different professions considered the same patient vignette. They found that psychiatrists tend to adopt a "medical model" of mental disorder. They tend to think that psychiatric disorders are medical disorders, and are appropriately treated by drugs. Nurses take a somewhat similar approach. In contrast, social workers usually adopt a social model. They think that mental disorders are caused by social stress, and are best treated by counselling or social interventions. A study by Bridget Hamilton *et al.* (2004) confirms these findings. Hamilton *et al.* examined how members of different mental health professions seek and obtain different information from patients admitted into acute psychiatric units. They found that nurses focus on the patient's immediate behaviour and interaction on the ward; psychiatrists sought to make a diagnosis as soon as possible, as a prelude to making treatment decisions; social workers would first try to find out where and how the patient lived, and what they normally did in an average day. Clearly the members of different mental health professions tend to operate within different paradigms.

A substantial literature examines communication within multidisciplinary mental health care teams. As such, looking at multidisciplinary teams is a good starting-point for assessing Kuhnian claims about incommensurability. Research looking at communication in multidisciplinary teams has found that, as Kuhn would expect, problems with communication regularly arise. In particular, many writers have noted that problems with communication often occur between health care professionals and social workers (Hiscock & Pearson 1999; Gulliver *et al.* 2002; Stanley *et al.* 2003). Many social workers consider there to be a "social work culture" that is different from the cultures of health care. Among other distinguishing features, this culture is said to place great value on client self-determination and so to contrast with the "more paternalistic culture of health professionals" (Peck & Norman 1999: 237). In the words of Pauline Gulliver *et al.*, between social work and health care there are "two different systems … different cultures … different languages" (2002: 365).

Not all the reported problems with communication arise for Kuhnian reasons, however. On occasion, great communication difficulties can arise between doctors and nurses. The theoretical views of these groups are similar so, following Kuhn, communication between them might be expected to be relatively easy. But often it is not. In her detailed study, *Conflicts in Care: Medicine and Nursing* (1993), Lesley Mackay examined doctor–nurse communication. She concluded that problems arose because of the difference in status between the professions. Doctors are well-educated, well-paid and trained to be confident in their decision-making abilities. Stereotypically, doctors are also male and middle class. Nurses have none of these advantages. In Mackay's study, communication problems arose because nurses did not feel able to speak up, and because doctors did not listen to them when they did. The timing of the empirical work for Mackay's study meant she was looking mainly at communication between non-graduate nurses and doctors. In the UK, new nurses now tend to be graduates. However, more recent research suggests that this has led to little improvement in communication between the two groups. Colombo *et al.* (2003) describe how psychiatrists continue to ignore the views of community psychiatric nurses, and how nurses consequently feel unable to speak their mind. This probably reflects the fact that nursing degrees are still low status compared with medical degrees. Here the basic problem is not that Kuhnian incommensurability prevents psychiatrists from understanding nurses. Rather, the problem is that differences in status mean that nurses do not speak and doctors do not listen. Differences in status restrict communication between different mental health professionals.[2]

Inter-professional rivalries caused by differences in status and working conditions limit communication between different types of professional, but there are also deeper reasons why those who work within different paradigms in the psych-sciences will tend to dislike each other. It is natural for those who work with mentally ill people to want their patients to get better, so when there is disagreement as to how patients should be treated, tensions are bound to arise. Practitioners will not merely think that those who work within different paradigms are wrong, but will view them as being a danger to patients or, at the very least, as a waste of valuable resources. Consider relations between biologically oriented psychiatrists and psychoanalysts, for example. Psychoanalysts and biologically oriented psychiatrists tend to disagree about who should be treated, and about what the outcome of treatment should be. Analysts have tended to prefer to treat intelligent patients suffering from neuroses. In contrast, drugs can be used to treat the very sick. Analysts value "insight", whereas biologically oriented psychiatrists want to get their patients back into the community, and preferably into work, as quickly as possible. These differences lead to trouble. Analysts have often dismissed drug cures as superficial. They have thought that drugs provide symptomatic relief only and may reduce a patient's motivation to seek deeper change. On the other hand, biologically oriented psychiatrists allege that analysts treat only rich and relatively healthy patients, and ignore those whose need is greatest. As a consequence, hostility arises on both sides.[3]

The members of distinct paradigms can also cultivate more subtle differences. Luhrmann found that in every hospital she visited there was an implicit dress code whereby "doctors looked like one another and emphatically not like nurses" (2000: 93). The biologically oriented psychiatrists she met also looked different from the psychoanalysts. In some cases they "adopt a style that seems deliberately to signal that they are not the tweedy, reserved psychoanalysts of their supervisor's generation … They pump iron, play squash … go drinking … talk quickly and loudly" (*ibid.*: 173).[4] Going further back, Arnold Rogow's *The Psychiatrists* (1971) documented in detail the extent to which analysts and psychiatrists differed in a multitude of respects. Compared with psychiatrists, analysts were more cultured and read more "high-brow" literature, and they claimed greater left-wing sympathies (although they spent a great deal less time treating poor patients). Together such differences of style and attitude mean that members of a particular professional group will tend to find it easier to talk to other members of their own group rather than to outsiders.

Even when individual members of distinct professional groups do attempt inter-paradigm communication they may find their efforts are discouraged by members of their "home" paradigms. One of Luhrmann's respondents started as an analyst but became increasingly interested in biologically based psychiatry. His analytic supervisor noticed his increasingly biological leanings and warned him, "People take up sides around here and you'll find yourself on the wrong side" (2000: 176). Rather like street gangs, the members of a scientific paradigm may jealously guard their numbers and territory.

We can conclude that many communication difficulties between mental health professions are caused by inter-professional rivalries and hatreds. When mental health professionals do not respect each other, or actively dislike each other, they are less likely to try to understand each other.

6.5 Coordination without full communication

So far, we have looked at reasons why communication between mental health professionals working within different paradigms might be difficult. However, clearly at least some communication occurs between groups: members of multi-disciplinary groups manage to coordinate at least some of their actions. In his important book *Image and Logic* (1997), Peter Galison provides a framework for thinking about when, how and to what extent communication between different paradigms might be possible. Galison's study looks at patterns of communication between theorists, experimenters and instrument-makers in high-energy physics. He describes how groups of scientists can coordinate their actions and beliefs to achieve a common goal, even though they may not be able to fully understand each other.

Galison draws on work by anthropologists who have examined how trade works between distinct cultures. Even when groups have very different world-views, and indeed very different understandings of the goods they wish to exchange, trade is still possible. Where the groups meet, "contact languages" spring up to enable the coordination of action. Pidgins are simple contact languages with a limited range of application. A pidgin might enable the exchange of buttons and buffalos, but is not complicated enough to meet all the language needs a human being might have. On occasion a pidgin may develop into a creole: a fully fledged language. Often this happens when children begin to grow up using the pidgin as a natural language and it thus has to develop to meet all human language needs.

The interesting thing about pidgins that are used to facilitate trade is that groups using the language can get by with a very limited understanding of each other. One group might think of coins as merely being useful tokens that one can exchange for food. Another group may attribute all kinds of mystical properties to money. Still, it can be agreed that a sack of flour, say, can be swapped for two coins. Similarly, Galison thinks that groups of scientists can develop contact languages to coordinate their actions, even though they have very different understandings of their work.

> Like two cultures distinct but living close enough to trade, they can share some activities while diverging on many others. What is crucial is that in the local context of the trading zone, *despite* the differences in classification, signification, and standards of demonstration, the two groups can collaborate .... (Galison 1997: 803)

Here I shall use Galison's ideas to discuss how inter-paradigm communication in the psych-sciences has been enabled by the creation of contact languages.

6.5.1 The DSM as a contact language

Perhaps the best example of a contact language in the psych-sciences is the DSM, which aims to list and describe all known mental disorders. The DSM has a long history, but here we need only concern ourselves with the editions since the DSM-III, published in 1980. The committee that created the DSM-III wanted it to be used by all mental health professionals. This goal was problematic as mental health professionals operate within numerous different theoretical frameworks, and there were fears that a DSM based on any one particular theory would alienate many practitioners. To avoid this problem, the DSM-III committee set out to base the DSM on no theory at all (American Psychiatric Association 1980: 7). Instead they aimed to produce a purely descriptive classification system that makes no use of hypotheses regarding aetiology.

One thing that can be said at the outset is that the DSM-III committee failed in its aim of producing a theory-free classification system. Consider the way in which many DSM diagnoses contain exclusion clauses. Let us take agoraphobia. This can only be diagnosed if the symptoms cannot be better explained by a major depressive episode, obsessive compulsive disorder, paranoid personality disorder or schizophrenia. These disorders trump agoraphobia because the pathological processes underlying them are thought to be more severe than that underlying agoraphobia. Quite clearly a theory of mental disorders is needed to support such judgements.

The DSM-III is not theory-free. However, to a large extent it has succeeded in only assuming theoretical claims on which there is broad consensus. Thus, although mental health professionals disagree on many points, as the DSM makes use of only those theoretical claims on which most agree, it can be used by most of them.[5] Like a contact language, the DSM works by getting practitioners to bracket off much of their knowledge when they use it. Thus, in many contexts a psychoanalyst and a biologically oriented psychiatrist mean very different things by "anxiety", but in the context of DSM-talk they know that only a pared down meaning is in play. A paper by Deborah Cabaniss, a psychoanalyst writing in 2001, nicely illustrates how the language of the DSM enables contact between psychoanalysts and biologically oriented psychiatry. Cabaniss discusses how she uses DSM criteria to determine whether her clients suffer from a constellation of symptoms that might be treated by psychoactive drugs. She herself remains committed to a psychoanalytic framework but is prepared to bracket out this knowledge when making treatment decisions. She writes, "The emphasis on careful diagnosis and phenomenology to guide treatment decisions does not, however, neglect the importance of understanding the meaning of the use of medication – it only moves it out of the sphere of decision making" (2001: 164). In other words, like a contact language, the DSM facilitates inter-paradigm communication by enabling professionals to bracket off much of what they believe for particular purposes.

In the light of the previous discussion of inter-group rivalries, it is worth noting that many professionals do not use the DSM through choice but because they are forced to. In the US, medical insurance companies will often only reimburse for psychiatric treatment if a patient receives a DSM diagnosis. A study of clinical and counselling psychologists revealed that although only 17 per cent considered the DSM to be a satisfactory classification system, 90.6 per cent used it; and 86.1 per cent noted that they had to use the DSM to obtain insurance reimbursement (Miller *et al.* 1981). Plausibly, contact languages prosper when external constraints force different groups to communicate.

6.6 Aiming for full communication across paradigms

The communication that is facilitated by Galison's contact languages is extremely limited. The contact language enables the coordination of action, but does so by bracketing off points of theoretical disagreement. What, however, if a scientist does not merely want to coordinate action with members of another paradigm, but wants to understand them? Maybe, for example, he or she wants to be able to judge which theory is best. How might it be possible to gain full understanding of another paradigm?

6.6.1 Multidisciplinary training

Sometimes multidisciplinary training is promoted as a solution to problems with communication (e.g. Colombo *et al.* 2003: 1569). The thought is that if mental health practitioners are trained to understand several different approaches to understanding mental disorder then mutual understanding between groups will be easier.

There are reasons for thinking that this approach is mistaken, however, and here I will suggest that multidisciplinary training does not enable inter-paradigm understanding. The problem is that plausibly the individual who has been trained to work within several paradigms just ends up being able to switch between them, but still cannot integrate them. This claim is most closely associated with Quine. In a famous thought experiment, Quine asks us to consider the position of the linguist who attempts to translate English into a radically different language, in his case "Jungle". Quine thinks that effecting such a translation will be problematic.[6] At one point he considers whether a bilingual might be able to overcome the difficulties associated with radical translation, and be able to translate between the languages while others fail. Quine suggests that the advantages of the bilingual speaker are limited. According to Quine, the bilingual will have to set about his task "much as if his English personality were the linguist and his jungle personality the informant; the differences are just that he can introspect his experiments instead of staging them" (Quine 1960: 71).

I suggest that the position of the bilingual speaker is analogous to the position of the mental health practitioner who has been trained in multiple paradigms. The bilingual can switch between languages. Similarly the practitioner trained in multiple paradigms will be able to switch between thinking in different ways. This claim is supported by Luhrmann's findings. The trainee psychiatrists she studied were trained in both analytic and biological approaches to mental disorder and could operate within both frameworks. Nonetheless, although Luhrmann's respondents could switch between frameworks they still had problems integrating the approaches. One of her respondents (a psychiatrist just out of residency) reported: "I attempt to integrate the two but it's more like I shift gears but it's a little jerky. I'm always shifting back and forth" (Luhrmann 2000: 238). In other words, multi-paradigm training can enable one to know what an analyst would think, and what a psychopharmacologist would think, but it does not enable one to integrate the two approaches to work out which is the better.

6.6.2 Direct patient contact

Kuhn believes that communication between scientists who work within different paradigms is problematic because the scientists see the world differently, they use terms with different meanings and they have different values. In an as yet unpublished paper, Krystian Burchnall (2006) has argued that case conferences play an important role in facilitating inter-paradigm communication in psychology. I think that Burchnall is right, and that inter-paradigm communication is possible when multiple practitioners have access to, and discuss, the same patient.

Psychoanalysts and biologically oriented psychiatrists rarely, if ever visit patients together. Here, however, I shall imagine that an analyst and a biologically oriented psychiatrist do jointly visit a patient in order to explore how their problems with communication might be overcome.

Perceiving the world differently

Kuhn argues that scientists who work within different paradigms will perceive the world differently. He claims this largely on the basis of experimental evidence regarding subjects looking at playing cards, electron tracks and so on. Plausibly, however, looking at human subjects is very different from making observations in other domains. Throughout evolutionary history human beings have needed to look at other human beings, whereas playing cards and electron tracks are recent phenomena. As such, we might expect people to be good at looking at people, and maybe not so good at looking at more recent stimuli.

Following on from this, I suggest that all human beings find certain human behaviours highly salient. If someone has smeared faeces over himself or is pulling out his hair then all perceivers will notice this, regardless of their theoretical training. Thus, our biologically trained psychiatrist and our psychoanalyst can be expected to make some common observations. On the other hand, other aspects of behaviour may be more subtle, and here differently trained practitioners may perceive different things. Their training will have made them alert to different aspects of the patient's behaviour, and they are likely to ask different sorts of questions and so to elicit different information. Suppose, though, that the analyst and the biologically oriented psychiatrist examine the patient together, and that they point out their observations to each other. Then will they perceive the same things? For the most part I suggest they will. To a large extent scientists belonging to different paradigms see different things because they look in different places and are alert to different things. Working together can rule out these sources of difference.

Still, a few differences in the perceptions of the scientists might remain. Plausibly, expert wine tasters can make discriminations that non-experts cannot make. Even with an expert guiding one's tasting, it might be the case that a trained palate can taste things that a normal person's cannot. Such sources of difference will plausibly be few and far between, but they may occur. Perhaps, for example, one practitioner has spent years working on the increased rates of speech that can occur in mania. This scientist has trained to discriminate rates of speech that the average listener cannot distinguish. He or she claims that a patient is talking somewhat fast; to the other scientist the rate of speech sounds completely normal. In such a case, I suggest that the best thing to do is simply to trust the observations of the more discriminating scientist (assuming that their perceptions meet standards of reliability, for example, they sort "quick speakers" and "normal speakers" into consistent groups). By such means the two scientists can ensure that they have the same evidence base to work from. When practitioners working within different schools have direct access to the same patients the communication problems that might be caused by varying perceptions can be overcome.

The meaning of terms

Kuhn argues that scientists belonging to different paradigms will talk past each other because even when they use the same words their terms differ in meaning. I suggest that there are two means by which such difficulties can be reduced to insignificance.

- *Nagel's suggestion*. In his 1971 paper "Theory and Observation", Ernst Nagel argues that the theory-ladenness of terms is often unproblematic in practice. According to Nagel, scientists with different theoretical orientations can often still mean the same thing by their observation statements. Although their observation statements are theory-laden, as long as the theories assumed by the observation statements do not include those theories about which the scientists disagree, their differing theoretical beliefs will not lead to any difference in meaning. Nagel's point is best made clear by considering an example. Suppose our psychoanalyst says to the biologically orientated psychiatrist, "Mr Smith has been crying". This is a theory-laden statement. It assumes, for example, that Mr Smith is a human being with mental states rather than a cunningly constructed robot, and that the liquid coming from his eyes is tears rather than sulphuric acid. Still, following Nagel, even if "Mr Smith has been crying" is theory-laden, the psychoanalyst and biologically orientated psychiatrist can mean the same thing by the statement. While many of their theoretical beliefs and assumptions will be different, many of them will be shared. As long as the beliefs assumed by "Mr Smith has been crying" are among those they hold in common, they should experience no problems in communicating.
- *Causal accounts of reference*. The meaning of some terms is given by their place in a theory, as Kuhn says. However, in other cases the meanings of terms can be fixed by links with the world. One can point at some item in the world, for example a new species of flower, baptize it, by saying something such as "Let's call this a Lesser Yellow Spotted" and then henceforth the name can be used to refer to all items of the same kind.[7] Often a "type specimen", that is a preserved organism, will be kept for reference, maybe

in the Natural History Museum in London, for example. "Lesser Yellow Spotted" then refers to all flowers of the same type as the baptized original. When the meaning of a term is fixed in such a way, all users of the term can talk about the same thing, regardless of their theoretical beliefs. One group of botanists may believe that lesser yellow spotteds are closely related to orchids and another think that they are not, but when they talk to each other these differences do not matter. Both groups are talking about plants that are of the same kind as the baptized sample.

I suggest that the meanings of terms for some psychiatric symptoms can be fixed by pointing at a prototypical example, in the same sort of way as can the meanings of names for biological species. Take, for example, the symptom of waxy flexibility. The limbs of a person displaying waxy flexibility can be placed into peculiar positions, and will be held for an unusually long amount of time. Symptoms such as this can be named via the baptism of a particular example. When a physician sees such a symptom for the first time he or she can baptize it – "Let us call this 'waxy flexibility'" – and then the term comes to refer to all symptoms of the same kind. I suggest that the case studies via which a symptom is first described can fix the names of psychiatric symptoms in much the same kind of way as type specimens fix the meanings of the names of biological species.

When the meaning of a term is fixed by pointing at an example of a kind, the fact that different theorists may have different beliefs about things of that kind is irrelevant. Regardless of their different beliefs, all speakers talk about the same thing.

When practitioners from different schools talk to each other, their terms will have the same meanings when *either* the term is theory-laden, but only with theoretical commitments that they share, *or* the term's meaning is fixed by pointing at samples in the world. Together terms of these types will give the practitioners some common language.

Differences in values

Those who work within different paradigms may have different values. In the mental health sciences almost everyone accepts that getting patients better is of key importance. However, even once this is agreed, practitioners working within different paradigms may disagree as to what constitutes improvement or recovery.

Consider differences between psychoanalysts and biologically oriented psychiatrists, for example. Analysts value "insight" and they tend to want their patients to achieve a higher level of functioning than before they became sick. Biologically oriented psychiatrists are more likely to aim to get their patients back into the community, and preferably into work, as quickly as possible. As a consequence, there can be disagreement as to whether a treatment has worked or not. A biologically oriented psychiatrist may consider a patient who lacks insight but has returned to work to be a treatment success, while an analyst would not.[8]

Those who work within different paradigms may disagree as to what constitutes a good outcome. However, such differences may be insignificant in practice, as increasingly mental health professionals are forced to assess outcomes on the basis of standards that are imposed by external bodies, such as drug approval agencies and the funders of mental health care. Take drugs trials, for example. The data collected in these studies must be acceptable to the bodies that approve drugs: the Food and Drug Administration (FDA) in the US and the Medicines and Health Care Products Regulatory Agency (MHRA) in the UK. These bodies have a history of accepting studies that measure outcomes via rating scales that measure changes in the symptoms associated with specific mental disorders (such as the Hamilton Depression Rating Scale). As a consequence, researchers designing drug trials use these rating scales, rather than alternatives that, for example, ask patients how much their quality of life has improved (Gilbody *et al.* 2003: 27).

Similarly, the bodies that fund mental health care can determine how outcomes will be measured. So, for example, the US Department of Veterans Affairs (VA) uses the Global Assessment of Functioning (GAF), to help evaluate the allocation and effectiveness of the mental health care it funds (Moos *et al.* 2002). Such a body has the power to make the professionals it employs comply with its demands.[9] Along the same lines, in the UK some National Health Service Trusts have tried requiring psychiatrists to collect data on patients using the Health of the Nation Outcome Scales (HoNOS) (Gilbody *et al.* 2003).

Scales such as the GAF or HoNOS can be seen as contact languages that enable professionals who work within different paradigms to discuss treatment outcomes. As with the DSM, externally imposed pressures force practitioners to use the language and they are able to communicate with it. Once again, the contact language works by forcing practitioners to bracket off points of disagreement for the purposes of communication. In the words of one of the respondents in Gilbody *et al.* (2003), "HoNOS although scientifically flawed is useful for bringing together all the members of the Multi Disciplinary Team" (*ibid.*: 50). When external bodies dictate the standards that will be used to assess treatments, differences in the values of those who work within distinct paradigms cease to be barriers to communication.

6.7 Conclusion

To summarize, in this chapter I have argued that the psych-sciences offer genuine examples of sciences where the existence of multiple paradigms within a sub-discipline is the norm. For philosophers, psychiatry thus offers an especially interesting case for considering Kuhn's claims. Kuhn claims that scientists working within different paradigms will have problems communicating. In most sciences this claim is hard to test, as multiple paradigms compete only during revolutions, but revolutions are rare and last only for a comparatively short time. In the psych-sciences, however, multi-paradigm sub-disciplines are the norm, and multi-professional teams force the members of different paradigms together. Psychiatry thus offers the ideal test case for working through Kuhn's claims about incommensurability.

In this chapter, I have argued that communication across paradigms in the psych-sciences is problematic, and is made harder by inter-professional rivalries and hatreds. However, although inter-paradigm communication is hard work it is possible: contact languages enable the coordination of action across paradigms, although they achieve this by bracketing off points of theoretical disagreement. In addition, I have argued that joint interaction with the world (as occurs when therapists together consider the same patient) can enable full communication across paradigms. I conclude that the communication that can occur across paradigms in the psych-sciences demonstrates that communication across Kuhnian paradigms is possible, although difficult.

This chapter also offers suggestions for mental health professionals. If I am right, then members of different paradigms who want to communicate can best achieve this by structuring their attempts in particular ways. Where contact languages already exist, they should be used. Where contact languages do not exist, they need to be created. Members of distinct paradigms who wish to communicate should also seek to maximize the time they spend together investigating relevant aspects of the world. In the case of mental health, this will generally mean that they need to interact jointly with patients.

7. Relations between theories 2
Reductionisms

Within psychiatry, theories at "different levels" can seek to explain and predict the same phenomenon. So accounts of depression are offered in neurochemical, sub-personal, personal, familial and societal terms. How do such theories fit together? Are they in competition, or might they all be true? What does it mean to say that one theory can be reduced to another?

In this chapter I, first, disentangle three distinct questions that reductionists might ask, and then go on to consider which reductionist theses, if any, are plausible in the case of psychiatry.

7.1 Three types of reductionism

At the outset we need to distinguish between three different varieties of reductionism:

- *Metaphysical reductionism.* A metaphysical reductionist claims that entities at a higher level are nothing over and above entities at a lower level. So, for example, a crowd is plausibly nothing more than a collection of people. Once the facts about the people and their positions are fixed, so too are facts about the crowd. Within psychiatry, the interesting question is whether the mind is anything over and above something physical. These debates are metaphysical. They have to do with the nature of reality.
- *Epistemic or explanatory reductionism.* An epistemic or explanatory reductionist holds that claims at one level can be reduced to claims at lower levels. So an epistemic reductionist might hold that the science of psychol-

ogy can be reduced to neurology, for example. This is an epistemic claim. It has to do with human knowledge.

- *Methodological reductionism.* A methodological reductionist holds that it is a fruitful strategy for scientists to attempt to explain phenomena by reducing them. Such attempts may not always succeed, but the methodological reductionist thinks that attempting reduction is a good method for scientists to follow.

Although these three types of reductionism are distinct positions, there are links between them. As we shall see, one's metaphysical view of the mind will affect whether one thinks that psychological theories can be reduced to neurological theories, for example. With these varieties of reductionism distinguished we can go on to consider what kinds of reductionism, if any, are plausible in the case of psychiatry. At least in the case of the mental, questions of metaphysical reductionism and epistemic reductionism are closely linked, and so we first consider these together.

7.2 What is the mind? Can theories about the mind be reduced to theories about the brain?

In the case of psychiatry, the big questions here are whether the mind is reducible to something at the physical level – brain processes, say, or behaviour – and whether theories in psychology can be reduced to theories in some more basic science. Here I shall not attempt to resolve the vexed question of the relationship between mind and brain. In this section I shall attempt only to outline a few of the possible positions and to explore the implications of adopting the different views for psychiatry.

In recent years there has been a fair amount of interest in the mind–body problem in psychiatry journals. In particular, Kenneth Kendler (2001; 2005) has published papers on the mind–body problem in the *American Journal of Psychiatry*. Here I shall use Kendler's work as a foil in developing my claims in this section. There are multiple possible views on the relationship between mind and brain, but we start by reviewing the four examined by Kendler: dualism, identity theory, functionalism and eliminative materialism. Considering these four views will enable us to get some idea of the possible accounts that are available, and also to consider how the account of mind that one adopts might have implications for psychiatric practice and research. Having examined these four views we shall then go on to look at one last account that Kendler does not discuss: Donald Davidson's anomalous monism. Anomalous monism is worth examining because it is one of the most sophisticated accounts of mind currently available, and is an example of a view that holds that although the mind is physical, psychological explanations cannot be reduced to explanations in a more basic science.

7.2.1 First account: dualism

Over the centuries many different accounts of the mind have been termed "dualist". Here we consider classical substance dualism, as advanced by René Descartes ([1641] 1968). The main motivation behind dualism is that minds are strikingly unlike all other known physical entities. Consciousness, subjectivity and intentionality are all special features of the mental. One question that we need to address is why it is that minds display these features but other things do not. Dualism supplies one possible answer. Dualists think that minds display special features because minds are made out of a fundamentally different kind of stuff than physical objects. The dualist claims that physical and mental things are different to the extent that the categories that apply to one type of substance simply do not apply to the other. For example, in the case of physical things it makes sense to ask what shape they are, how big they are and so on. In the case of mental states such questions lack application: to ask about the shape or colour of my beliefs simply does not make sense.

The main problem faced by dualism is that it seems metaphysically extravagant. If we can give an adequate materialist account of the mind this would be preferable because we will then end up with a simpler and more unified overall world-theory. If the mind is the brain, or patterns of behaviour, or some such, then this will fit far better with a broadly materialist worldview. This being said, many philosophers hold that all materialist accounts of the mind fall into difficulties and that dualism is thus the only viable option (e.g. Chalmers 1996). Dualism thus remains a respectable position in the philosophy of mind.

Within the psychiatric literature a number of misconceptions can be found concerning dualism. Three in particular are worth discussing here.

Misconception 1: psychiatric research has shown that dualism is false

Various writers in psychiatry have claimed that psychiatric research has shown that dualism is false. So Kendler states: "It is time for the field of psychiatry to declare that Cartesian substance dualism is false" (2005: 434; see also Miresco & Kirmayer 2006). Unfortunately, these authors do not cite the particular research that they take to refute dualism. One can only assume that they are referring to neuroscientific research that shows that subjective experiences are correlated with particular types of brain activity. I shall argue that such evidence is insufficient to disprove dualism.

One must accept, of course, that advances in contemporary neuroscience have been astounding. Still, all such research shows is that there are *correlations* between some subjective experiences and properties of the brain. While the details of this claim can be filled out better than ever before, it is important to note that the claim itself is nothing new. Descartes himself knew that physical events and mental events are causally connected: if you put your hand in the fire it hurts; if you put a sword through someone's skull this may affect their ability to speak. One can be a dualist about the mind and make sense of all neuroscientific findings so long as one holds that among human beings there are reliable correlations between brain events and mental events. So long as such correlations hold, one can say that brain scans can give one good reason to think that someone is in pain, for example. For the dualist, what one sees in the brain scan is not itself pain, but is a reliable marker for pain. This is good enough for brain scanning research to be worthwhile. Similarly, as a dualist, one can accept that, say, antidepressants help with depression. One need only hold that the physical effects of the antidepressant reliably bring about a change in mood. Once again, the challenge posed by such mind–brain correlations is fundamentally nothing new: Descartes knew that alcohol changes mood. I conclude that neuroscientific findings, no matter how cutting edge, do not show that dualism is false.

Misconception 2: dualism is required for a belief in life after death

Many people associate dualism with religious beliefs. When we die our bodies are burnt or rot, and so if one believes in life after death it is tempting to think of the mind, or soul, as something quite distinct: another kind of substance that carries on once the body is gone. However, the claim that one needs to be a dualist to believe in life after death is not quite right. One can be a materialist and also believe in life after death in at least two ways. First, one might believe in a bodily resurrection, so our bodies and minds both exist after death. Secondly, one might think of the mind as being something abstract, like the information encoded on a CD. The information on a CD cannot survive without being on any disk at all, but it can be moved from one disk to another. Similarly, one might think that the collection of mental states that makes up one's mind might be realized by another system after one's body has died. Thus one does not need to be a dualist to believe in life after death.

Misconception 3: dualism is needed for free will

Finally, some have claimed that one needs to be a dualist in order to believe in free will (Miresco & Kirmayer 2006). The problem of free will is that there seems to be a tension between two plausible claims: that human beings can decide how they act; and that all events in the world are governed by physical laws. How can these two claims be compatible? Consider the case where I am short of cash and so steal an ice cream from a shop. How can it be true that I am responsible for my action and could have done otherwise, and yet also be true that my taking the ice cream was entirely predictable, given the physical position of the various particles that make up my body?

The problem of free will is difficult, and will not be solved here. All I aim to do here is to make it plausible that adopting dualism about the mind does not help much with the problem. The dualist claims that the mind is distinct from the body. As such, it is a possibility that mental events will not be governed by natural laws. (Note that this is only a possibility; many dualists have actually thought that physical and mental events will be lawfully linked). If mental events are not governed by natural laws then maybe truly spontaneous thought is possible. Maybe my desire to take an ice cream was not determined by my genes and upbringing, but arose freely. However, now we must ask about the actual act of picking up the ice cream. This is a physical event and will be governed by physical laws. Although dualism may open up the possibility that my thoughts may be free, it does not help when it comes to considering my actual physical actions. My intention to steal may be spontaneous, but the actual theft remains predictable by physical laws. Thus dualism does not help in resolving the problem of how I might be responsible for taking the ice cream and yet the action be entirely predictable. Adopting dualism will not help with the problem of free will.

I conclude that dualism is compatible with all neuroscientific findings, and with the fact that psychoactive medications can change mental states. One can thus adopt dualism without this causing any problems for psychiatric research. Within the psychiatric literature dualism is sometimes presented as being a dead theory. But it is not. There are still reputable philosophers of mind who are proud to be considered dualists, for example, David Chalmers. Turning to the question of whether psychological theories can be reduced to theories in neuroscience, we can note that dualists will not think that such reductions will be possible. They hold that the mental is something beyond the purely physical, and thus mental states will have properties that cannot be captured by physical theory.

7.2.2 Second account: identity theorists

Sometimes neurosurgical procedures are carried out while patients are conscious. This enables the surgeon to talk to the patient and to obtain information regarding the progress of the operation. In *Psychosurgery in the Treatment of Mental Disorders and Intractable Pain*, Walter Freeman and James Watts ([1942] 1950) report on a conversation between Freeman and a patient during a lobotomy. The conversation runs as follows:

> Freeman: "What's going through your mind?"
> Patient (after a long pause): "A knife" (*Ibid.*: 116)

That psychosurgery results in mental changes clearly illustrates that the mind and the brain are closely connected. Depending on the bits of the brain that are removed, characteristic mental changes result. But is the patient literally right to say that a knife is going through his mind? An identity theorist will say that the patient is right. The knife going through his brain is going through his mind. And, if a surgeon cuts out $5cm^3$ of the patient's brain then he has cut out $5cm^3$ of the patient's mind.

Identity theories are most closely associated with U. T. Place (1956) and J. J. C. Smart (1959). They claim that each type of mental state is identical with a type of brain state. The example commonly given is that pain might turn out to be identical with C-fibres firing, say. Identity theorists see such claims as scientific hypotheses. They think that pain might turn out to be identical with C-fibres firing in the same kind of way as water turned out to be H_2O. Identity theorists think that the mind is the brain in the same kind of way that lightning is electricity, and sound is compression waves in the air.

If the identity theory turns out to be correct it is easy to understand why psychoactive drugs can affect mental states: in altering brain chemicals such drugs alter mental states. (Note that, as we saw, the dualist will also accept that drugs change mood but on their account it is harder to see exactly how psycho-physical causal processes are supposed to work). Similarly, on the identity theory it is easy to see why psychiatrists are interested in brain imaging studies. The identity theorist can look at such work and suggest that at some point in the future it will advance to the stage where we shall be able to literally see individual mental states. In the psychiatric literature such a view is clearly expressed in Eric Kandel's 1998 paper "A New Intellectual Framework for Psychiatry". Kandel looks forward to the day when brain imaging eventually allows psychiatrists to *see* that their patients are getting better. He expects that, "As the resolution of brain imaging increases, it should eventually permit quantitative evaluation of the outcome of psychotherapy" (Kandel 1998: 460).

The identity theory holds that the mind is the brain. If this is correct then psychological theories can be expected to be reducible to neurological theories. Instead of talking about pains we could switch to talking about the neurological properties that are identical with pain, in the same sort of way that physicists can talk about mean kinetic energy instead of temperature.

However, despite its attractions, there is one big problem for the identity theory. Identity theorists claim that each type of mental state is identical with some type of brain state. So, pain might be identical to C-fibres firing and a belief that chocolate is the best flavour ice cream might be identical to neurons 5c and 6f lighting up. But what if beings with different types of brain can be in the same mental state? Hilary Putnam (1975) asks us to consider octopuses. Octopuses are intelligent – they can solve mazes and unscrew jar lids to get food in jars – but they are very unlike us. Both an octopus and a human being can be in the same kind of mental state; maybe both intend to reach for something. When the human being reaches out their arm their brain controls the action. But when an octopus reaches out its arm, things work rather differently. In a gruesome study, German Sumbre *et al.* (2001) removed an octopus's arm and then applied electrical impulses to the arm; they found that it moved out much as it would if still connected to the octopus. They took this to show that "The basic motor program for voluntary movement is embedded within the neural circuitry of the arm itself" (*ibid.*: 1845). If they are right then this means that when human beings intend to move their arm activity occurs in their brains, but when an octopus intends to move its arm some of the activity is in its arm. In this case there cannot be a brain state that is identical to an intention to move: the human being and octopus are in the same mental state, but neurologically they are very different.

Even if we stick to human beings it seems that a particular mental state can be realized by different types of brain activity. Some people who suffer brain damage recover to a greater or lesser degree. They may have a stroke that destroys part of their brain, and then after a while other parts of their brain take over the functions of the destroyed areas, and they get better. In a 2002 study, Valeria Blasi *et al.* compared normal subjects with people who had recovered from strokes that had damaged the language areas of their brains. Blasi's team first measured the two groups' performance while they performed a word-stem completion task. Participants saw three letters at a time and were asked to say a word that began with those three letters. For example, if they saw the letters "COU" they might say "cougar". Brain images from stroke patients revealed several differences. Language areas damaged by the stroke were not active during the language task. However, areas on the right side of the brain opposite the damaged areas on the left did become active during the task. This means that Person A might think "Cougar starts COU" and Person B might also think "Cougar starts COU" but completely different parts of their brain can be activated in each case.

These examples make it plausible that beings with very different brains can be in the same mental state. This means that mental states can be *multiply realized*. A state can be multiply realized when physically different states can be functionally equivalent. Examples of things that can be multiply realized are mousetraps and computer programs. Mousetraps can take various designs and be made of different materials, but, as they all catch mice, they all count as mousetraps. Similarly computer programs can be run on different types of machines. As mental states can plausibly be multiply realized, mind–brain identity theories are often considered to be untenable. This pushes us to consider our third account of the mind: functionalism.

7.2.3 *Third account: functionalism*

We looked briefly at functionalism about the mind in Chapter 4, but it is probably worth reminding ourselves what functionalists claim. Functionalists take the multiple realization of mental states seriously. Functionalism is an account of mind that specifically aims to accommodate the idea that physically quite different beings can be in the same mental state. The functionalist claims that mental states should be characterized functionally, in terms of their characteristic sensory inputs, behavioural outputs and links with other mental states. Functionalists often suggest an analogy with computing. Computer programs are paradigmatic examples of functionally defined entities because the same program can be run on physically very different systems. Functionalists encourage us to think of the mind as being the software that runs on the hardware of the brain.

To take an example, let us consider how a functionalist would characterize a particular belief, say a belief that it might rain. Such a belief has:

- characteristic sensory causes, for example, people generally form this belief after watching the weather forecast and hearing that it is going to rain, or by seeing clouds;
- characteristic behavioural consequences, for example, in combination with a desire to avoid getting wet, it causes people to carry umbrellas or to stay inside; and
- characteristic links with other mental states, for example, if someone was planning a barbecue then it will tend to produce disappointment, but if they are concerned about their lawn being too dry then they may be relieved, and so on.

The functionalist claims that any state that fulfils this characteristic functional role is a belief that it might rain. One thing to notice is that in characterizing the belief in this way, the functionalist makes no claims at all about what kind of stuff is realizing the functions: it might be a brain state; it might be a state of some electronic gadgetry in a robot head; or it might be a state of green gunge in a Martian. As long as it is related to sensory inputs, behavioural outputs and other mental states in an appropriate type of way it counts as a belief that it is going to rain. Functionalists do not care what realizes a mental state. One consequence of this is that while functionalism is compatible with materialism (i.e. one can consistently be a functionalist and a materialist) it is not, in itself, a materialist theory. The functionalist does not make any claims about what minds are made of. Conceivably one could have minds made out of appropriately organized soul stuff.

If functionalism is adopted as an account of mind one implication is that we should expect human beings to be vulnerable to two types of mental disorder.

Some would be caused by problems with the hardware of the brain. Others would be caused by problems in the "software" of the mind.

Functionalism and explanatory reductionism

If functionalism is correct, then this has implications for the question of whether psychological theories can be reduced to theories in a more basic science. In his paper "Special Sciences (or The Disunity of Science as a Working Hypothesis)" (1974) Jerry Fodor argues that it will not be possible to reduce theories that describe and explain the behaviour of functionally defined kinds. Functionally defined kinds can be multiply realized, and Fodor argues that this means they cannot be reduced. Take money, for example. Money is a functionally defined kind and can be multiply realized. Anything that can be used as a unit of exchange counts as money, and money can be made of physically very different things: gold, silver, paper, salt and so on.

Now consider the laws of economics. These are laws about money. Could these laws be reduced to laws in some more basic science, say physics? Fodor argues that they could not. The problem is that bits of money can be physically very different. If we were to begin reducing the law we would get something like this: "When small silver disks of such and such a diameter, or small pieces of paper 10cm by 5cm, or such and such electric pulses on the internet, or …". We would have to continue the list to include all the things that have ever been used as money. But even then we would not be finished because scientific laws are supposed to tell us what is possible as well as what is actual. So we would also have to include in the list all the types of physical thing that could ever be used as money. But this list would be infinite: the law could never be completed. This shows that it is impossible to reduce a law about money to a law of physics.

With regard to money, we can now see that it is both consistent and sensible to be a metaphysical reductionist but not an epistemic reductionist. Following Fodor we can accept that laws about money cannot be reduced to laws in physics; thus we will not be epistemic reductionists in this area. Still, we should accept that all bits of money are ultimately made of physical stuff – there is no irreducible "money substance" in the world – as such we will be metaphysical reductionists regarding money.

If we adopt functionalism as a theory of mind, Fodor's argument can be applied to psychological laws. If pain can be multiply realized and there are laws regarding agents' responses to pain, it will not be possible to reduce such laws to laws in neurology. However, as we saw in Chapter 4, the implications of Fodor's argument for psychiatry are limited. Multiple realization implies that not all pain will be neurologically alike: Martians and some unusually wired human beings may realize pain in odd ways. Still, it is consistent with this to think that normal human pain may be C-fibre activation, while Martian pain may be something else.[1] While the functionalist is committed to the claim that pain might be realized by all sorts of odd physical systems, they can still claim that all normal human pains may be physically similar and there might be reducible laws governing such pains.

Problems with functionalism

Although functionalism has attracted many adherents, it is not without problems. Functionalists claim that mental states can be defined purely in terms of sensory inputs, behavioural outputs and interactions with other mental states. However, problems arise when one considers how one should specify the sensory inputs and behavioural outputs. If one specifies them in terms of normal human sensory inputs and human behaviour, then one risks chauvinism about the mind. One will end up saying that only beings that can have normal sensory inputs and can manifest normal human behaviour have minds. This is a problem because the very point of functionalism was to allow for the possibility that many different types of being – advanced robots, intelligent aliens, octopuses – might have minds.

On the other hand, one might seek to specify the sensory inputs and behavioural outputs in more abstract terms. Here one would just end up having a map showing the functional links between these different inputs and outputs. The problem now is that one risks being far too liberal. Maybe all kinds of things that clearly are not minds can be functionally organized like minds. In a famous thought experiment, Ned Block (1978) asks us to consider the population of China. According to Block, it so happens that there are about as many people living in China as there are neurons in the average head. Now, suppose the government of China is persuaded by philosophers of mind to try the following experiment. You are asked to read a passage from a book and then to write a report on it. During this time the Chinese government monitors your brain and keeps track of what each of your neurons does. Then some Chinese people act as your eyes did, taking in data regarding the passage from the book. Others act as your neurons did, passing messages from one to another. Finally, some Chinese people act as your hands did, producing exactly the same report as you did. For a while, the population of China is functionally equivalent to your brain, but does the population of China have the same mental states as you did? Some functionalists will bite the bullet here and say that in such a situation China does have a mind. But many people think this is the wrong thing to say. They think that the population of China could not have a mind and that this example suggests that there are deep problems with functionalism.

To sum up, functionalism is a theory of mind that is designed to accommodate the multiple realizability of the mental. If functionalism is correct then, as Fodor argues, it will not be possible to reduce the laws of general psychology to laws in a more basic science; the desires felt by a human being and those felt by a robot will not have anything physically in common. Nevertheless, although the desires of robots will be physically very unlike my desires, maybe all normal human desires are physically alike. If this is the case then it may still be possible to reduce psychological laws if we restrict our attention to the case of normal human beings. As a theory of mind, functionalism has its defenders, but it faces difficulties. In particular, specifying the inputs and outputs associated with functionally defined mental states in such a way as to avoid falling into the problems of chauvinism or liberalism will be difficult, if not impossible.

7.2.4 Fourth account: eliminative materialism

Eliminative materialists think that mental states do not exist. Compared with the other accounts we have looked at, eliminative materialism has only a fringe following among philosophers, but it has been much discussed within psychiatry and so will be reviewed here.

Eliminative materialism has most famously been proposed by Paul Churchland (1981). His argument for eliminativism starts from the assumption that we should seek a scientific theory that will describe and explain everything in the world. All our common-sense notions should, eventually, be replaced by scientific ones. The eliminative materialist has a vision of the state of human knowledge in which we currently, to put it crudely, believe in too many types of things. Our list of the different things that we think exist is too long and too motley; currently it includes things as diverse as tables and electrons, beliefs and wars. As knowledge progresses we will be able to shorten our list of our ontological commitments. There are two ways in which we can shorten our list: entities may be reduced or eliminated. The difference between elimination and reduction is best illustrated with an example. The example is whimsical, but the best I can think of to convey the point.

Consider possible ways the Loch Ness Monster theory might develop. Every year scores of people go to Loch Ness in Scotland in the hope of seeing the legendary Loch Ness Monster. Let us imagine two possible scenarios where researchers succeed in accounting for the Loch Ness Monster sightings:

- Scenario 1: scientists discover that a specimen of a giant sea eel lives in Loch Ness.
- Scenario 2: scientists find that they can explain each and every monster-sighting. Some can be explained as sightings of shoals of small fish swimming in formation; some turn out to be nothing but strangely shaped tree branches; in some cases it turned out that the observers were drunk and had overactive imaginations.

In the first case the Loch Ness Monster theory is *reduced* to the giant sea eel theory. Here it is sensible to say such things as "It turns out that the Loch Ness

Monster is a giant sea eel". In this case, although the monster turns out to be not quite what we expected, there is something that can be identified with the Loch Ness Monster. In the second case the Loch Ness monster is *eliminated*. Here we would say, "It turns out that the Loch Ness Monster does not exist". In this case there is no one thing that can be identified with the Loch Ness Monster. To generalize, entities are eliminated when we are forced to conclude that they do not exist: witches, caloric and ether have been eliminated from our world-theory. On the other hand, entities are reduced when we conclude that they are identical with another type of entity: heat has been reduced to mean kinetic energy.

What determines whether a theory is reduced to another or eliminated? Roughly it depends on how badly wrong the theory is. In the first scenario the Loch Ness Monster theory could be reduced to Giant Sea Eel theory (and the monster reduced to the particular eel) because if there were a giant sea eel in Loch Ness, the Loch Ness Monster theory would not be all that far off track. In the second scenario, the Loch Ness Monster would simply be eliminated because it would turn out that the Loch Ness Monster theory was just too wrong for it to make sense to say that the monster existed.

Returning to the mind, we have already discussed some accounts whereby the mind is reduced to the brain: mind–brain identity theories are an example. In contrast, eliminative materialists claim that there are no such things as beliefs or desires, or, to put their claim slightly differently, they think that minds should be eliminated. Eliminative materialists claim that our common-sense theory according to which human beings have various beliefs and desires must be eliminated because it is just too wrong to be reduced to neuroscience or any other scientifically respectable account of the mind.

Churchland claims that our common-sense folk psychology according to which people have beliefs and desires is a shockingly bad theory. He condemns it thus:

> what we must say is that FP [folk psychology] suffers explanatory failures on an epic scale, that it has been stagnant for at least twenty-five centuries, and that its categories appear (so far) to be incommensurable with or orthogonal to the categories of the background physical science whose long-term claim to explain human behaviour seems undeniable.
>
> (1981: 76)

As examples of mental phenomenon that folk psychology fails to explain he cites "the nature and dynamics of mental illness, the faculty of creative imagination, or the ground of intelligence differences between individuals" (*ibid.*: 73). Churchland claims that folk psychology has not progressed since the times of the ancient Greeks. Furthermore he cannot see how common-sense claims regarding beliefs and desires can be made to fit with the findings of neuroscience. For these reasons Churchland thinks that folk psychology should be rejected. Once common-sense folk psychology has been abandoned, Churchland expects neuroscience to supply us with completely new concepts for explaining and predicting each other's behaviour, and for expressing our own inner life.

In the psychiatric literature, Kendler (2001) discusses eliminative materialism. His paper has been influential, but he manages to confuse eliminative materialism with both straightforward materialism and epiphenomenalism (*ibid.*: 991–2). It is important to note that eliminative materialism is distinct from both these positions. Eliminative materialists think that mental states do not exist, while materialists can accept mental states so long as they are material (so identity theorists are materialists but not eliminative materialists, for example). Epiphenomenalism is a variety of dualism according to which mental states are real, and have physical causes, but themselves have no physical effects. Because epiphenomenalists accept the existence of mental states this position is also distinct from eliminative materialism.

The basic difficulty with eliminative materialism is that it is an extremely radical position that demands that we completely revise out current ways of thinking. Most people are strongly committed to the claim that they and the people they know have minds. It seems unproblematic for me to make multiple claims about my mental states: I *desire* a nice cup of coffee; I *believe* that my plants need watering; I *intend* to go to the cinema tonight; and so on. Similarly you can also reel off lists of your mental states. The eliminative materialist claims that all this talk of minds and mental states is literally nonsense. Adopting eliminative materialism would require radical changes not only to our ordinary ways of thinking, but also within psychiatry. If eliminative materialism is the correct account of the mind then all talk of mental states must eventually be abandoned. For most, this would imply too radical a departure from our present practices for eliminative materialism to be an attractive position. As such, eliminative materialism remains a marginal position in the philosophy of mind.

7.2.5 Fifth account: anomalous monism

Donald Davidson was one of the most influential, but also one of the most difficult, twentieth-century philosophers of mind. His account of mind has been much discussed in the philosophy of psychiatry, and is one of the most sophisticated accounts of mind currently available.

Davidson (1980a) puts forward a view of the mind that he calls anomalous monism. Davidson claims that all individual mental events are brain events, but he also denies the possibility of reducing psychological laws to physical laws. As such, Davidson is an example of someone who is a metaphysical reductionist but not an epistemic reductionist.

Davidson argues that psychology cannot be reduced by arguing that there cannot be strict psycho-physical laws. As such, the claims of psychology cannot be reduced to the claims of neurology. In arguing against the possibility of psycho-physical laws, Davidson asks us to consider how we attribute mental and physical states to an agent. Here we shall first consider mental states.

The mental according to Davidson

Davidson claims that we cannot attribute beliefs and desires to an agent one by one; rather, we have to attribute them as a set. I shall explain why Davidson thinks this is the case in two ways.

- *Mental state attributions are open to revision.* Our judgement of what other agents believe can be endlessly modified as we learn more about their other mental states. To illustrate, suppose a woman goes over to a tap and turns it on. What might we conclude from this? We probably conclude that she wants a drink of water and believes that water will come from the tap. But suppose we then hear her say "I'll need to take a sample of this". Then we might conclude that she believes the water has been contaminated and a sample needs to be taken. Can we stop here? No, because we might then learn that the agent believes herself to be in a play. Then we would conclude that the she is just pretending to take a sample. The point is that when we attribute beliefs and desires to an agent we always have to be open to the possibility that we may have to revise them in the light of evidence concerning the agent's other mental states. Thus, we cannot attribute mental states one at a time.
- *The principle of rationality.* Davidson thinks that mental states have to be attributed as a set because they must accord with the principle of rationality. When we ascribe intentional states (e.g. beliefs and desires) to an agent we follow certain principles of rationality. These principles ensure that the total set of intentional states that we ascribe to an agent is as rational and as coherent as possible. For example, suppose we are trying to ascribe intentional states to someone who says "I love Tony Blair and I hate him". We will tend not to ascribe the inconsistent intentional states of both loving and hating Tony Blair to the person. Rather, we will search for some interpretation of the person's utterances whereby we can attribute a consistent set of intentional states to her: maybe when she says "I love Tony Blair and I hate him" she means "I love some aspects of his personality and hate others".

  When we attribute intentional states to an agent we try to attribute a set of intentional states that are as rational and as consistent as possible. Davidson thinks that this requirement of rationality and coherence is of the essence of the mental, that is it is constitutive of the mental in the sense that it is exactly what makes the mental mental. Or, to put it another way, a being whose beliefs were not largely rational and coherent would not count as a believer at all. As we have to attribute consistent beliefs to a believer, we cannot attribute beliefs one by one because we may have to revise our attributions in order to make them consistent with later utterances.

The physical according to Davidson

Now consider how we attribute physical states to someone. We simply have to weigh them or measure them or whatever and then we can conclude that, for example, "Fred weights 80kg". We can attribute physical states on a one-by-one basis. Once we have weighed Fred we can conclude that he weighs 80kg and any evidence that comes up later concerning his other physical states cannot force us to revise this attribution. Regardless of his height, hat size or inner leg measurement, we can continue to assert that Fred weighs 80kg. Characteristically, attributions of physical states can be made on a one-by-one basis.

As physical states can be attributed one by one whereas mental states have to be attributed as a set there can be no psycho-physical laws. We can see why this is so using a *reductio* argument. A *reductio* argument is one where we assume some premises for the sake of argument, show that an absurd conclusion follows and thus conclude that the initial premises should be rejected. Davidson asks us to suppose, for *reductio*, that there are laws that connect beliefs with brain states, for example, a law that states that any agent with neurons 5f and 6g firing believes that Tony Blair is a great man. If there were such a law, then when we looked inside the agent's brain and saw those particular neurons firing we would be able to attribute the belief to the agent on that basis. We would be able to attribute beliefs on a one-by-one basis. But, now we run into a problem: if we could attribute beliefs one by one then they would no longer be constrained by the rationality principle. But, since beliefs necessarily accord with the rationality principle, this would mean that any such states would not be beliefs. Therefore, Davidson concludes, there can be no psycho-physical laws. As Davidson himself puts it, "nomological slack between the mental and the physical is essential as long as we conceive of man as a rational animal" (1980a: 223).

Davidson is not an epistemological reductionist, but he is a metaphysical reductionist. He thinks that each mental event is also a physical event. His view is called anomalous monism. Anomalous monists hold that ultimately there is only one kind of stuff in the world: physical stuff. However, they think that mental talk – our talk of beliefs, desires, hopes and all the rest – cannot be reduced to physical talk. We could not give up talking about mental states and just talk about brain states. This is a consequence of there being no laws that link kinds of mental event with kinds of physical event. The physical events that are identical with instances of some kind of mental event need have nothing in common. Thus we could not stop talking about people hoping to catch the last train, for example, and start talking of people being in a particular brain state, because the brain states that are identical with instances of hoping to catch the last train need have nothing in common and so we will not be able to invent a new word that will pick them out from all the other brain states.

A note on Davidson on irrationality

Davidson's argument that there can be no laws linking physical and mental events made crucial use of his principle of rationality. It was part of Davidson's argument that beliefs and desires are essentially rational. This means that we have to attribute consistent and coherent beliefs to agents. And this means that beliefs can only be attributed as a set and not on a one-by-one basis. In contrast, we can attribute physical states one by one. This means that there can be no laws that link mental and physical events. The principle of rationality – that beliefs and desires are essentially rational – is a crucial premise for this argument. Davidson's whole argument for anomalous monism only goes through if the principle of rationality can be upheld.

However, although human beings are often rational there seem to be cases where they are not. Before considering cases of irrationality that pose a threat to Davidson's project, we should first dispense with some cases that might be described as cases of irrationality but that actually cause him no problems. We might want to say that a desire to take heroin is irrational. The disadvantages of becoming a heroin addict outweigh the possibility of heroin-taking being a pleasurable experience to the extent that we may find it hard to empathize with someone who wants to take the drug. Similarly, a fear of spiders or a sexual fascination with shoes may strike us as irrational. Beliefs may also be irrational in the same kind of way, for example, someone might have an unfounded belief that crystals can be used to cure people. Irrationality in this sense does not pose a threat to Davidson, however. Davidson's principle of rationality states only that an agent's beliefs and desires must be consistent and coherent. The principle tells us how beliefs and desires must be related to each other, not what they should be. A person may have a weird belief or desire but, as long as it is consistent with their other beliefs and desires, their intentional states may still satisfy the principle of rationality.

The principle of rationality is only threatened by cases where an agent has beliefs and desires that are inconsistent or incoherent. Let us consider a commonplace example. Suppose someone admits that there is a negligibly small chance of winning the lottery. Certainly, they say, the chance is so small that it is not enough to balance the hassle of buying the ticket. Then they go out and buy a ticket, and later they turn on the television especially so that they can see which numbers come up. In such a case we feel pushed to attribute inconsistent beliefs to the person. We feel pushed to say that the person both believes that he has no chance of winning the lottery and yet also believes that it is worth buying a lottery ticket. Such cases appear commonplace. And, if human beings often have intentional states that are neither rational nor coherent this poses a serious threat to Davidson's principle of rationality.

In his paper "Paradoxes of Irrationality" (1982), Davidson considers how he can revise his account so that it can cope with such cases of irrationality. Davidson asks us to consider a simple case of irrationality. To adopt his example, suppose that a woman's son has been arrested for some offence. She very much wants him to be innocent, and this leads her to believe that he is innocent. This is a simple case of wishful-thinking. That the woman's desire that her son be innocent leads her to believe that he is innocent is easy enough to understand, and yet if the entire explanation for her belief is that she wants it to be true her belief is irrational. After all, her wish to have a belief is not evidence for the truth of the belief; her desire does not justify her belief in any way.

Davidson claims that such a case of irrationality may be characterized as being a case in which there is a mental cause that is not a reason. The woman's desire causes her belief, but is not a reason for holding the belief. Davidson's admission that in some cases mental states cause other mental states but are not reasons for them leads him into difficulty. For Davidson, mental states must be rational or they do not count as mental states at all. How does Davidson get out of this difficulty?

Davidson's way out is to point out that there are other everyday cases in which mental states can cause other mental states and yet not be reasons for them. Suppose I want you to notice me. I wear a pair of flashing devil's horns when I go to the bar that I know you will be in. The flashing horns attract your attention and you look at me. My desire that you notice me causes you to look at me, but my desire is not a reason for your action (you might not even know that I wanted you to look at me).

Having considered such examples Davidson concludes that "Mental phenomena may cause other mental phenomena without being reasons for them, then, and still keep their character as mental, provided cause and effect are adequately segregated" (1982: 300).

Davidson suggests that this example can provide us with a model for dealing with non-reasonable mental causes as they occur in a single mind. The trick is to think of the mind as consisting of several quasi-independent sub-structures. The different sections of the mind can be thought of as acting on each other in a way analogous to the way in which different people interact. This claim forces Davidson to revise his principle of rationality. Rather than claiming that the intentional states of an individual must be consistent and coherent, he now claims only that the intentional states of each section of the mind must show a large degree of internal rationality and consistency.

If Davidson's revised principle of rationality can be maintained then his argument for the anomalism of the mental will go through just as well as it would if his original principle were viable. A consequence of adopting either principle is that beliefs must be attributed as a set. As physical states can be attributed on a one-by-one basis this means that there can be no psychophysical laws.

If the mind consists of several independent parts then we can understand how a person can harbour inconsistent beliefs and how their mental states can interact as non-reasonable causes. Different sections of a mind can have inconsistent beliefs in the same way that the beliefs of two people may be inconsistent. The mental states of one section of the mind can cause mental states in another section in the same way that the mental states of one person can cause the mental state of another.

This way of thinking about things enables us to deal with the examples of irrationality that we considered earlier. To return to the lottery ticket example, we can say that one part of the mind believes that there is a negligible chance of winning the lottery and that there is no point to buying a ticket, but that another part of the mind believes that there is a chance of winning the lottery and that buying a ticket is worthwhile. It is worth noting that the model of mind proposed by Davidson has important similarities with that proposed by Freud. For both thinkers, the mind contains a number of semi-independent structures, and these have mental attributes such as thoughts and desires.

Another note on Davidson: the implications of his claims are limited

In his 2003 *British Journal of Psychiatry* paper "Psychiatry and the Human Sciences", Mark Turner uses Davidson to argue that:

> mental symptom-concepts, particularly those of minor mental illness and personality disorder, have broadly rational conditions of application; they relate to individuals' other beliefs, desires and action in a normative way that cannot be captured by a theory that is formulated in a physical vocabulary. (2003: 473)

I think that Turner overstates the case here, and that the implications of Davidson's claims for psychiatry are limited. In so far as Davidson's argument works it applies only to those mental states that can be rational. As Davidson himself puts it, his arguments are "limited in application to branches of psychology that make essential reference to 'propositional attitudes' such as belief, desire and memory, or use concepts logically tied to these, such as perception, learning and action" (1980b: 240).

If Davidson is right our beliefs and desires must be governed by the principle of rationality. But there are many other types of mental states to which rational norms will not apply. Pains, nightmares and feelings of panic, for example, will not be governed by the principle of rationality, and thus even if one buys into

Davidson's argument, psychological theories about such states might be reduced to physical terms.

In addition it is questionable whether states such as delusional "beliefs" act in ways that accord with the principle of rationality. Delusional beliefs behave differently from normal beliefs. Normal beliefs are revisable in the light of new evidence: if I believe that your dog is vicious and then you show me that it is friendly, I will revise my belief. This is part of what it means to say that normal beliefs are governed by the principle of rationality. In contrast, delusions are retained even when there is good evidence that they are false, and their links with other mental states may also be odd (so in some cases deluded people fail to act on their deluded beliefs, for example). To the extent that delusions do not act as normal beliefs, they will not be governed by the principle of rationality and Davidson's argument will not apply to them either. Thus, even if Davidson is right, a good part of psychiatric theory may turn out to be reducible to the theories of some more basic science.

7.2.6 Summary of accounts of the mind and implications for psychiatry

We have looked at five different accounts of the mind. The different accounts are summarized in Table 7.1. It is worth noting that in addition to the pure accounts of mind discussed here, "hybrid" accounts are also possible. One might, for example, be a functionalist about beliefs and desires, an identity theorist about emotions, and an eliminativist about intuitions and acts of will. Furthermore, accounts of mind different from those discussed here are also available. However, the accounts of mind surveyed here are sufficient to illustrate the range of accounts that are available, and to enable us to discuss some of the implications for psychiatry that will follow from adopting one account of the mind rather than another.

Of the five accounts we have considered, in my opinion dualism, identity theory, functionalism and anomalous monism are viable theories. Although, as we have seen, these accounts face difficulties, there are philosophers of mind who are currently working on and refining these views. Eliminative materialism has a far smaller following.

The most important implication that I wish to draw from this survey of accounts of the mind is that one does not have to be a dualist in order to think that the mind is real. Identity theorists, functionalists and anomalous monists also believe that the mind is real. Identity theorists think that the mind is real and is identical with the brain. Functionalists think that the mind is real and is functionally defined. Anomalous monists think that each particular mental state is identical with a brain state, but that there are no strict laws governing the mental. Only eliminative materialists deny the existence of the mind. This point has been missed in several recent papers in psychiatric journals. For example,

Table 7.1 Summary of accounts of mind

Account	Claims	Can psychology be reduced to neuroscience?	Advantages	Problems
Dualism	Mind is a different stuff	No – psychological properties cannot be captured by physical theories	Explains why minds are different from other things	Does not fit well with a physical worldview
Identity theory	Mental states are identical with brain states	Yes – psychological properties just are neurological properties	Fits neatly with physical sciences	Runs into problems with the possibility of multiple realization
Functionalism	Mental states are functionally defined	Multiple realization means that a reduction of "general psychology" cannot be achieved, but species-specific reductions are not ruled out	Can accommodate multiple realization	Depending on how inputs and outputs are defined, risks falling into chauvinism (e.g. denying that paralysed people have minds) or liberalism (claiming that China has a mind)
Eliminative materialism	Mental states do not exist	Psychology is nonsense and should be eliminated	Claimed to fit with expected future scientific findings	An unattractively radical view
Anomalous monism	Mental states are brain states, but psychology cannot be reduced to neuroscience	Talk of rational mental states cannot be reduced, but Davidson has nothing to say about non-rational psychological states	A non-dualist account that goes some way to explaining what is special about the mental	Not discussed here (see Heil & Mele 1993: pt 1).

Miresco and Kirmayer (2006) found that clinicians tended to use psychological explanations when they reasoned about disorders such as drug addiction or personality disorders. They worry that clinicians continue to think of some forms of mental illness as being especially "psychological", in defiance of research that, they claim, has shown that dualism is false. Here Miresco and Kirmayer are doubly confused. First, as argued earlier, psychiatric research has not shown, and cannot show, that dualism is false. Secondly, all materialist accounts of the mind – with the exception of eliminative materialism – provide room for the legitimacy of psychological talk. As long as one steers clear of eliminative materialism, talk of mental states is safe.

Depending on the account of mind one adopts, one will expect there to be different varieties of mental illness. Most notably, functionalists think of the mind as being analogous to the software that runs on a computer. They will expect that there will be two possible types of mental illness. While some disorders may result from "hardware" problems with the brain, others may be caused by problems with the "software" of the mind.

With the exception of eliminative materialism, all the theorists we have examined accept that the mind is real and has causal powers. All can thus expect there to be mental disorders that have psychological causes. Even mind–brain identity theorists allow this. Suppose I see terrible things and suffer from post traumatic stress disorder. The identity theorists can accept that the images processed by my brain have led to nightmares and so on. On their account, my perceptions and nightmares just are types of brain state, so it is not surprising that they have causal effects. All theorists also accept that the physical is real and can affect the mental. If I poison my brain with drugs all theorists will expect this to affect my mind. Even dualists can allow for this, as they accept that physical events can bring about mental changes.

The different theorists have different views about the prospects of reducing psychological theories to neuroscientific theories, and before we go on it is worth reminding ourselves of the arguments here. As we have seen, Fodor argues that theories about multiply realized entities resist reduction. If mental states are functionally defined then this would imply that a universal psychology (i.e. one that applied to all kinds of minds) could not be reduced. Nevertheless, it may still be possible to reduce psychological theories of more restricted scope. Even if Martians and robots have mental states that are realized in physically diverse ways, it may still be the case that normal human mental states are physically alike and thus reducible. In so far as psychiatry seeks only to account for the mental states of human beings, the implications of Fodor's argument for psychiatry will thus be limited.

Davidson also argues that psychology cannot be reduced. Again, I think the implications of his argument for psychiatry are restricted. Davidson's argument only applies to propositional mental states that are rationally related. Much of psychiatry deals with mental states that are either non-propositional (feelings of panic, anxiety) or are not rationally linked with other mental states (delusions). Thus, even if Davidson's argument is accepted, theories about such psychological states might be reducible to theories at a lower level.

So as long as one rejects dualism, projects within psychiatry that aim at reducing theories at the psychological level to theories at lower levels may yet prove successful.[2]

7.3 Methodological reductionism

The final question that we should consider is methodological. Is it a good idea to try to reduce things if you want to explain them? Those who think that seeking reduction is a good tactic can be termed "methodological reductionists". It is important to note that methodological reductionism is a comparatively weak position. The methodological reductionist claims not that all attempts to reduce phenomena will be successful, but merely that attempting to reduce them is a reasonable way to proceed. Typically, methodological reductionists will seek to justify their stance by considerations drawn from the history of science. The history of science indicates that sometimes reductions can be successful, and that even when attempts fail much can be learnt in the attempt.

Still, although methodological reductionism is a very weak thesis, at least in certain quarters methodological reductionism has a bad reputation. Many writers think that seeking reductionist explanations is somehow politically suspect. For a particularly clear example of such worries consider the following:

> The real problem with reductionism, though, is that as a way of looking at human beings it is both negative and misleading ... We need to look at explanations on a social level, as well as on an individual one ... the fact that reductionist arguments comfortably avoid questions like this is one reason for their popularity among the very right-wing sectors of society. (Hayes 1995: 16–17)

I think that seeking reductionist explanations is frequently justifiable and need not commit one to reactionary political claims. Reductionist explanations can be useful, because sometimes they give us a true account of why people behave in certain ways. Suppose, for example, that Steve is thrashing around on the floor, and we want to know why he is doing this. And, let us suppose that in this case Steve is thrashing around because he is having an epileptic fit. Explaining thrashing in terms of fits (and then in terms of brain processes) is a reductionist strategy. It is also the right strategy to adopt in this case. The reductionist explanation enables interventions that will make things better. Once Steve has been diagnosed as suffering from epilepsy, he can start taking drugs that will control his condition.

Nor need we restrict reductionist explanations to non-intentional behaviours (such as fitting). Suppose I go to pick up my friend at the airport and that she unfairly blames me for her flight delay. I am about to complain about her ingratitude, but then I reflect that she has been on an overnight flight and has not eaten for hours. Now I know that people frequently turn nasty when they are tired and hungry, and so I give her some food and let her sleep, and she becomes nicer. Once again this is a reductionist strategy. In effect I am explaining my friend's meanness in terms of physiological processes. Here too, though, the approach is justified. Often food rather than rational argument is the best remedy for irritation. There is nothing dehumanizing about recognizing that human beings are also biological animals.

All this being said, sometimes reductionist explanations do seem out of place. In his book *Crime and Disease* (1973), Anthony Flew discusses a young man who had shot his girlfriend nine times at point-blank range. His defence team argued that he was insane and did not understand what he was doing. Under questioning the defendant refused this explanation. Over and over again he was asked whether he had really meant to kill his girlfriend. Finally, he replied, "I fired to blow her fucking head off. How many times do you want me to tell you?", and then explained his motives for the attack (*ibid.*: 90). Here seeking to explain the defendant's actions using a reductionist explanation does indeed seem inappropriate. I suggest that the reason why reductionist explanations are out of place here is that in this case they do not explain the phenomenon very well. Explaining the defendant's actions in terms of motives yields a better explanation than does explaining his action in terms of illness and so to say that he was overcome by a flood of brain chemicals is dehumanizing.

I conclude that sometimes we are able to find good reductionist explanations (i.e. reductionist explanations with explanatory power) and that such explanations can be useful for guiding effective interventions. There is nothing wrong with looking for reductionist explanations, and it is reasonable to be a methodological reductionist. What we need to be wary of is imposing reductionist explanations in situations where they fail to explain phenomena as adequately as do higher-level explanations. There is nothing wrong with good reductionist explanations; it is only bad reductionist explanations that should be avoided.

7.4 Conclusion

To summarize, at the metaphysical level, within psychiatry the big question is whether the mind is anything metaphysically over and above the physical. We saw that there are various accounts of the mind on the philosophical market. Despite the claims of some writers, psychiatric research has not disproved dualism and it is still an open question whether the mind can be reduced to the brain. In any event, as long as one rejects eliminative materialism, mental states, whether reducible or not, will be real and talk of psychological states will be safe.

At the level of theories, the important question is whether psychological explanations can be reduced to neurological explanations. This question is distinct from the metaphysical question about the nature of the mind. One can be a materialist about the mind while also thinking that psychological theories cannot be reduced to theories in a more basic science. Fodor and Davidson both give arguments that might persuade one to adopt such a position. The arguments of Fodor and Davidson are widely accepted. However, I have argued that the implications of their arguments for psychiatry are limited, and that projects within psychiatry that aim to reduce psychological theories to theories at a lower level may prove successful.

Finally we considered methodological reductionism. I argued that methodological reductionism is a weak and reasonable position. Writers who argue that reductionist projects are in general politically dubious are mistaken.

8. Managing values and interests 1
Psychiatry as a value-laden science

Traditionally the aim of science has been to discover the truth about the world. The aim of psychiatric theory has, if anything, been even more ambitious, in so far as it has not only tried to discover the truth about mental illness, but also to use this knowledge to treat mental disorders, and so to make the world a better place.

Unfortunately, despite these noble objectives, when one looks back through history, the results have been disappointing. Considering scientific theories in general, the pessimistic induction is well known: when we look back at the history of science we see a long succession of rejected theories. The best scientists have been wrong over and over again. Given that current scientists are no cleverer than their predecessors, the odds are that our current best theories will also turn out to be wrong. Turning specifically to psychiatry, the evidence of history tells a yet grimmer tale. When we look back at psychiatric theory we see a long succession of theories that have not only been false, but have also been biased against the least powerful members of society.[1] What has gone wrong? That is, how has psychiatric theory tended to be wrong and biased against the least powerful? And, how might we make things better?

In this chapter, I shall consider the extent to which various types of value-ladenness might account for the poor track record of past psychiatric theory. Psychiatry has been accused of being value-laden in a multitude of different ways. In this chapter I tease out the various ways in which psychiatry might be value-laden and I consider which kinds of value-ladenness should reduce our faith in psychiatric theory and how any problems caused by value-ladenness might be overcome.

Before getting down to addressing these issues, however, clarification on a number of points may be helpful. First, I need to distinguish psychiatric research from psychiatric practice (although this distinction will not be watertight). At the level of practice, psychiatry is clearly affected by value judgements at every turn. Perceptions of neediness and worthiness affect who is diagnosed, and whether and how they are treated. This is not at issue; rather, here we shall be exclusively concerned with the question of whether values affect the scientific findings arrived at by researchers in psychiatry.

To give us a more precise definition of value-ladenness we can take it that to say that a science is value-laden is to say that the theories developed have been shaped by the values of the scientists. In other words, if a science is value-laden, then in that area scientific communities with different value-commitments can be expected to produce different scientific results. Groups of right-wing as opposed to left-wing scientists, or feminists versus male-supremacists, could be expected to produce different scientific findings.

To keep this discussion grounded, I shall consider these questions by looking at case studies drawn from articles that examine race and mental illness published in the *American Journal of Psychiatry* between 1844 and 1962. 1844 is when the *American Journal of Psychiatry* (then called the *American Journal of Insanity*) starts. These are papers from long ago, but focusing on these articles has several advantages. First, it enables me to follow the development of entire scientific debates in a way that would not be possible if I focused on more recent arguments. In the nineteenth and early-twentieth centuries most papers written by psychiatrists in the US were published in the *American Journal of Psychiatry*. As such, by reading through successive volumes it is possible to trace the way in which a debate unfolds. In contrast, with the exponential increase in scientific papers and proliferation of journals that occurred during the twentieth century, tracking entire debates in more recent psychiatry would be a fearsome undertaking. Later in this chapter I shall argue that it is important to focus on research programmes rather than individual papers if we are to understand the effects of value-ladenness, and so being able to trace entire scientific debates is important to me. Secondly, looking at old papers makes it easier to spot the values that shape research. This is because it is easier to spot the influence of values when those values are foreign to us than when they are values that we share. Thirdly, papers from the *American Journal of Psychiatry* have the advantage of accessibility. Most universities have access to this journal and papers back to 1844 are available in electronic form, so readers who wish to read the papers discussed here will be able to find them. These points made, focusing on late-ninteenth- and early-twentieth-century papers also carries problems with it. Possibly psychiatric science is no longer as shaped by values now as it was then. To address this concern, in each case where I identify in my case studies a variety of value-ladenness where it is not obvious that such value-ladenness will still be a problem, examples will also be given from contemporary research.

8.1 Introduction to the case studies

Before I outline the debates concerned with race and mental illness to be found in the *American Journal of Psychiatry* between 1844 and 1962, a terminological note is necessary. In describing the debates I shall use the terms for racial categories used by the participants. This is because the terms at times carried highly specific meanings, which would be lost if other terms were used. For example, in debates over the 1840 census, when participants spoke of "coloured" people they meant people whose female ancestors were presumed to be black slaves, and whose male ancestors were a mixture of black slaves and white slave owners. Translating such usages would lose the specific meanings of such terms, and so has not been attempted. With this in mind, we can go on to sketch the three debates to be found in the *American Journal of Psychiatry.*

8.1.1 The 1840 census

Four papers discuss the 1840 census (*American Journal of Insanity* 1844; 1851; Jarvis 1852; O'Malley 1914). The 1840 US census contained statistics on the numbers of "insane and idiots" divided by race. Moreover, as the coloured population in some states were known to be almost exclusively slaves, while those in other states were free, the incidence of mental illness among slaves and free coloured people could be compared. The initial statistics offered some highly surprising results. They suggested that rates of mental illness among slaves were far lower than those among free coloured people or white people. According to the census, rates of mental disability among free coloured people were ten times greater than among slaves (Deutsch 1944: 472). At the extremes, among coloured slaves in Louisiana only 1 in 4,310 was reported to be idiotic or insane while "every fourteenth [free] colored person in the State of Maine is an idiot or lunatic" (*American Journal of Insanity* 1851). Not surprisingly, such findings were enthusiastically received by pro-slavery groups. The pro-slavery politician J. Calhoun told Congress: "Here is proof of the necessity of slavery. The African is incapable of self-care and sinks into lunacy under the burden of freedom. It is a mercy to him to give him the guardianship and protection from mental death" (Wood 1885: 11, quoted in Deutsch 1944: 473).

Within the *American Journal of Psychiatry*, a lively debate concerning the interpretation of the statistics ensued. Did the Southern climate better suit coloured people? Were there mistakes in the census? Was slavery itself protective of mental disorder? Eventually a consensus was reached that the initial statistics had been misleading and that slavery does not offer protection from mental illness. The most likely explanation for the errors was considered to be that white pauper lunatics had mistakenly been entered into the columns for coloured lunatics. The columns of the census were very long, and the headings were thus far above where numbers were entered, so such mistakes could easily be made (*American Journal of Insanity* 1844; Jarvis 1852; Pasamanick 1962). However, although most authors agreed that the census findings were faulty, assertions that slavery protected slaves from mental illness continued to surface. As late as 1914 Mary O'Malley could write, "It is conceded by all who are familiar with the facts that insanity in the colored race has increased extensively since they acquired freedom" (1914: 317).

8.1.2 Mental illness among immigrants

Ten papers examine rates of mental illness among immigrant populations (Ray 1849; Ranney 1850; Salmon 1907; Ferris 1909; May 1913; Swift 1913; Rosanoff 1915; Dawes 1925; Malzberg 1935; 1936). These papers ask whether there are higher rates of mental illness among immigrants from certain countries. This debate occurred at a time when there was vast immigration into the US and the national mix of immigrants was changing; before 1900 most immigrants to the US came from Ireland, Germany and Scandinavia and after 1900 immigrants increasingly came from southern and eastern Europe. Furthermore, US mental hospital populations were rapidly increasing. At the practical level, papers that examined links between place of nativity and mental illness were linked to questions of immigration policy. If mental illness particularly affected persons from particular countries then immigration from those countries might be limited.

Eventually a consensus was reached that differences in rates of mental illness between immigrants and native-born people do not reflect intrinsic biological differences in susceptibility to mental illness but can be explained by differences in the age distribution of the populations and environmental factors.

8.1.3 Mental illness among different racial groups

Nine papers consider whether mental illness varies with racial group (O'Malley 1914; Bevis 1921; Wagner 1938; Ripley & Wolf 1947; Stevens 1947; St Clair 1951; Schermerhorn 1956; Wilson & Lantz 1957; Pasamanick 1962). This final debate goes on for a long period of time. The first paper on this topic was published in 1914 (O'Malley) and the debate continues throughout the period under study. Early papers (O'Malley 1914; Bevis 1921) claim that coloured people suffer from high rates of mental illness and that the psychoses from which they suffer are different from those that afflict white people. The authors attribute these differences to inherent biological differences: they claim that coloured people are at a lower evolutionary stage and thus break down differently. Later papers (Wagner 1938; Ripley & Wolf 1947; Wilson & Lantz 1957) continue to find higher rates of mental illness among negro people (in papers from 1921 on "colored" is replaced by "negro"), but these differences are now attributed to sociological factors: poverty, racism and so on. Finally, Pasamanick (1962) claims that there is little difference in rates of mental illness among different racial groups, and that if anything the white population might be more prone to mental illness (unlike earlier studies, Pasamanick counted not only the populations of state mental hospitals but also included the predominantly white populations of private and VA facilities).

Using examples from these three case studies, in the next section I shall show that psychiatric theory can be value-laden at every stage of scientific enquiry.

8.2 Varieties of value-ladenness

The articles drawn from the *American Journal of Psychiatry* illustrate how psychiatric science can be shaped by values at every stage of enquiry:

- picking the research area;
- formulating hypotheses to be tested;
- assessing evidence;
- presenting findings; and
- using findings.

The varieties of value-ladenness that I discuss here are not intended to be exhaustive; plausibly there are also other ways in which values can affect psychiatric research. Rather, they are chosen to be sufficient to show that psychiatric research can be affected by values in multiple ways and at multiple stages of enquiry. To make it plausible that the varieties of value-ladenness that I identify affect current psychiatric research and not just research from the late-nineteenth and early-twentieth centuries, whenever possible I will also give up-to-date examples of how value-ladenness continues to cause problems.

8.2.1 Picking the research area

It should come as no surprise that research tends to be directed at questions of concern. Research has to be funded and money will be directed at problems that are perceived to need solving. Furthermore, scientists themselves are likely to share the concerns of their society. As an example of the ways in which research comes to be directed at topics of current concern, consider the research looking at rates of mental illness among immigrants from different countries in the period 1900–1930. Interest in this topic was clearly linked with questions of immigration policy.

For a more contemporary example, Patrick Bracken and Patrick O'Sullivan (2001) discuss the lack of research into the health problems of people of Irish origin within the UK. Irish people form the largest migrant minority in the UK and also suffer from exceptionally poor mental health. Despite this, little research has looked at the health problems of the Irish. Far more work has looked at the problems faced by black and Asian immigrant groups. Bracken and O'Sullivan suggest that this is because Irish people – as a white ethnic group – fail to fit into the black and ethnic minority agenda.

Values lead researchers to direct attention at certain areas but not others. Epistemically one might be tempted to suppose that such value-ladenness is not too much of a worry. Truths will still be found (although they will be a subset of total truths). So we shall end up knowing things about black people but not Irish people, say, and while this may be a shame (or perhaps an advantage) for the Irish, at least truths are still being discovered. I think such a view would be overly complacent, however. When certain areas are investigated and others are not, then one can end up with a distorted view of an area. So, turning to a present-day example, more research funds have been spent investigating drug-based cures for mental illness than other types of therapy. One overall effect of this is to give the impression that drugs cures are in general more effective, although this might not be true.

8.2.2 Formulating hypotheses to be tested

Values are also involved when researchers formulate hypotheses for investigation. Depending on the researcher's outlook, different hypotheses will seem worth investigating. So, for example, in 1907 Thomas Salmon thought it worth exploring whether Jews suffer from higher rates of mental illness. Investigating this question was difficult – statistics recorded the nationality but not the religion of psychiatric patients – so Salmon had to go to great lengths to obtain data on Jewish rates of mental illness. Salmon's investigations were particularly focused on Jewish people. Neither Salmon nor anyone else bothered looking at whether rates of mental illness differed between, say, Baptists and Methodists. Here the hypotheses under investigation were clearly affected by the values of researchers. Jews appeared to Salmon to be a potentially problematic population.

8.2.3 Assessing evidence

So far the varieties of value-ladenness we have considered have been rather obvious. The ways in which values can affect the assessment of evidence are more subtle and more interesting. Values play a role when evidence is assessed for at least four reasons.

(i) Selecting a subject population

Although it does not come out very clearly in the particular papers under study, values are involved when psychiatrists decide which people count as suffering from mental disorder. Psychiatry is concerned with mental illness. However, as argued in Chapter 3, whether someone is mentally disordered or not is a value-laden question. A state only counts as a mental disorder if it is bad for the person with it. As such, only people who are considered to be in a bad way are deemed suitable subjects for psychiatric research. This can mean that over time the subject population studied by psychiatrists can shift, for example, the rates of mental illness recorded in the early-twentieth century counted homosexuals among the mentally ill. When different values mean that different researchers select different subject populations this is important because when different subject populations are studied different conclusions will be reached.

On a related note, studies have found that the diagnoses that are given to patients depend on their race and sex. Interpreting such studies is frequently difficult, as it is often unclear whether differences arise because the prevalence of mental disorders varies in different populations, or because psychiatrists see the same symptoms differently. In a 1988 study Marti Loring and Brian Powell attempted to get around these difficulties by asking psychiatrists to diagnose case reports that differed only in the race and sex of the patient. They found that the diagnoses given depended on the race and sex of both the patient and the psychiatrist in complex ways. To take one example, they found that 57 per cent of white male psychiatrists diagnosed one case as suffering from schizophrenia when the patient was said to be white, but 70 per cent diagnosed schizophrenia when the patient was black. The results from black male psychiatrists were even more striking. Here only 14 per cent diagnosed the white patient as schizophrenic, while 92 per cent selected this diagnosis for the black patient. Clearly the diagnoses that psychiatrists give depend not only on their patients' symptoms, but also on the value-laden expectations of the psychiatrist. When values lead psychiatrists to diagnose patients differently this will clearly affect psychiatric research findings.

(ii) Values and the Quine–Duhem problem/experimenters' regress

We briefly came across the Quine–Duhem problem, also known as the experimenters' regress, in Chapter 1. The problem is that experimental results and statistics rarely speak for themselves; rather, they have to be interpreted. Once a "raw" result or statistic has been collected scientists decide whether and how that result should be interpreted. This decision will be shaped by their prior beliefs and expectations. Investigators will look for correcting factors until they achieve a result that is in line with that that they anticipated. This point can be made clearer via an example.

In his 1907 paper "The Relation of Immigration to the Prevalence of Insanity", Salmon reported that "in 1906 forty-six per cent of the whole number of patients admitted to the New York State Hospitals were of foreign-birth, while the foreign-born population was but twenty-six per cent of the whole population of the State" (1907: 54). A debate followed concerning the interpretation of these data. In particular, researchers argued over whether these figures indicated that foreigners were more disposed to mental illness. In answering this question the statistics could be dealt with in at least four ways:

1. Accept the raw data at face value. Conclude that foreigners are twice as disposed to mental illness as natives. This option is taken by May (1913: 435) and Dawes (1925: 450).
2. Correct the data for age. Immigrants are mainly young people and this should be taken into account. So far immigrants have only displayed the illnesses of adolescence. As the immigrants age they will also suffer from the illnesses of old age. One can then draw the conclusion that foreigners are actually even more disposed to suffer from mental illness than the raw figures indicate. This option is taken by Salmon (1907: 61).
3. Correct the data for age. Immigrants are mainly young adults and include few children. Children tend not to suffer from severe mental illness. Once this is taken into account, the rates of mental illness among immigrant populations can be revised downwards. Foreigners are less likely to suffer from mental illness than the raw figures suggest. This option is taken by Swift (1913: 145).
4. The raw rates of hospital admissions for the foreign-born should be corrected for age (as in option 3). They should also be corrected for place of residence. Mental illness is more common among those who live in towns than those who live in the country, but foreigners are disproportionately urban. The extra stress experienced by immigrants should also be taken into account. After these corrections one can conclude that "There is no evidence to show that there is a greater proneness towards mental disease in the foreign-born than in the native population" (Rosanoff 1915: 57). Similar conclusions are drawn by Malzberg (1935: 627; 1936).

How does the scientist know how to adjust the results? Basically, what we see is that scientists adjust the result so that it fits in with their prior beliefs and expectations. Those who expect mental illness among foreigners to be higher search for reasons why the figures should be adjusted upwards. Those who expect no differences find ways of adjusting them downwards.[2]

(iii) Values and testimony

To a great extent psychiatric research relies on testimony. Researchers generally have to rely on others (assistant staff, relatives, patients) to tell them how the patient is doing. As such, questions arise as to who can be considered a reliable witness. Looking back through psychiatric research papers it is clear that a hierarchy of witnesses has often been in place. At the top of the hierarchy come psychiatrists, then assistant staff, followed by relatives and "respectable" patients. "Unrespectable" patients come at the bottom of the hierarchy of witnesses. This hierarchy has clearly been shaped by social assumptions.

In the papers I have been examining, the differential value placed on different types of witness is vividly brought out in papers concerned with mental illness among coloured people. In a particularly nasty example, O'Malley discusses the problems of relying on the testimony of coloured people in her "Psychoses in the Colored Race". She comments that "in collecting facts ... one encounters great difficulties, owing to the inaccuracy of their statements, which are at times more or less unreliable" and continues, "The colored are secretive by nature as well as by cultivation" (1914: 313).

Although nowadays rarely expressed in such offensive terms, the idea that there is a hierarchy of witnesses continues to play a role in current psychiatry. Consider, for example, the responses to Cathy Wield's book *Life after Darkness: A Doctor's Journey Through Depression* (2006). Wield's book is excellent in many ways, but for now I want to note only that reviewers and the publishers of the book have thought it important to emphasize that Wield is a doctor. Note that Wield is not a psychiatrist and this is not a book about how her views of mental illness have been altered by personal experience. Rather, stressing that Wield is a doctor seems to be important because it is taken to establish her reliability as a witness. An anonymous reviewer in the *Emergency Medicine Journal Supplement* (2006) writes, "Because this story is written by a doctor there is a general pragmatism running through it; many failings are accepted and understood but just as many are questioned and rightly so". Once decoded, I take it this translates to something like "Wield is a doctor and therefore worth listening to" (and, at least implicitly, those psychiatric patients who lack MDs are not).

As another example, consider how slow psychiatrists have been to allow patients to rate the severity of their own symptoms. Observational scales have traditionally been used to measure the severity of manic symptoms (so psychiatrists have observed rates of patient speech, irritability and so on). However, it turns out that manic patients can reliably rate their own symptoms: they can say whether it is true or false that they are sleeping less, talking more, feeling more irritable and so on (Bräunig *et al.* 1996). Similarly, patients with depression can reliably report the severity of their symptoms (Zimmerman *et al.* 2004). Given that mania and depression have long been known, how could it take psychiatrists until the 1990s to discover that depressed people know whether they have been waking up early in the morning? Why is it that the fact that some psychiatric patients can be reliable witnesses regarding their own symptoms was overlooked for so long? The most likely answer is that psychiatrists "simply do not trust [their] patients as observers" (Healy 1990: 120). Social assumptions about trustworthiness have led psychiatrists to assume that "crazy" people cannot be reliable witnesses.

(iv) Values and baselines: assumptions regarding normal bodies and minds
Often researchers assume that the "normal" is similar to themselves. Bodies and minds that differ from this "norm" then come to be viewed as deviations. The best known examples of such tendencies come from the biomedical sciences where the "normal" body has frequently been assumed to be male. So, for example, until recently clinical trials regularly used only male subjects, in part because womens' oestrous cycles were considered to distort results (Schiebinger 2003).

Similar assumptions can be found in the papers under study here. When discussing rates of mental illness, rates among the white population tend to be taken as the "normal" baseline. When different populations suffer from different rates of mental illness this is then interpreted as either an "excess" above the "natural" rate, or conversely as evidence of "under-representation". Such phrasing clearly reveals that the normal mind is assumed to be a white mind.

8.2.4 Presenting findings

As is well known, the language used to present findings is frequently value-laden, so it is good to be "normal", "high-functioning" and so on, and bad to be "psychotic" or of "below average intelligence". Plausibly, at least in the human sciences, it is not practically possible to create a value-free language. Attempts to do this have repeatedly failed. Here one need only consider the history of the changing terms used to describe people with learning disabilities. As each new term is introduced it quickly becomes as stigmatized as the term it replaces. While once schoolchildren called each other "mongs" and "morons" now they call each other "special".

When thinking of the ways in which language can be value-laden, the use of metaphors is particularly interesting. The metaphors in which research is couched tell the audience how to conceptualize the findings. They not only provide the reader with information but also tell them what to feel and think about it. For example, in discussions of mental illness and immigration the flow of mentally ill immigrants was likened to pollution (or in one case typhoid) seeping into a water source (Dawes 1925: 450; *ibid.*: 465 for Salmon's comments). The message is clear: the mentally ill immigrant is hereby presented as a massive threat who must be vigilantly guarded against.

8.2.5 Using findings

Finally, values clearly influence the use to which research findings are put. The clearest examples of this are the numerous cases in which research findings that are unwelcome to those who commissioned them are simply ignored. Often research is commissioned by parties who are not interested in discovering the truth about some question but who merely want to use the rhetorical power of science to justify decisions that have already been made on other grounds. For example, politicians continued to assert that the 1840 census figures showed that slaves suffered from lower rates of mental illness even when psychiatrists had reached a consensus that these findings were faulty. In the words of one Congressman: "It was too good a thing for our politicians to give up. They had prepared speeches based on it, which they could not afford to lose" (Wood 1885: 12–13, quoted in Deutsch 1944: 478). When research findings fail to fit in with political strategy they can simply be disregarded.

8.3 Comparison with other sciences

It is worth noting that other sciences are plausibly value-laden in the same sorts of ways as psychiatry. Let us take examples from botany and zoology. Values have clearly been involved at the stage of choosing research areas: much research has served the needs of empire (Browne 1996), or agriculture, for example. Values have been involved when evidence is assessed: various groups of people have been considered unreliable witnesses in natural history, and so observers who happened to be working class, female or amateur have frequently been sidelined (Secord 1996). Evidence has been interpreted so as to fit in with researchers' prior values. For example, the expectation that women should be sexually passive has led observers to interpret female organisms as manifesting such behaviour, and furthermore this observed passivity has then been used to justify the claim that such a state is natural for women (e.g. Haraway 1989). Values have been involved in the presentation of findings; the rhetorical links between talk of the threats posed by "exotic" or "alien" species and those posed by "alien people" have been well documented (see e.g. Helmreich 2005). Finally, values affect the use that is made of research findings. Consider, for example, the ways in which data on fish stocks are used to set fishing quotas. Depending on the politics of the time, such information may guide policy or be ignored. While psychiatric research is shaped by values so too is research in other areas.

8.4 What can be done?

We have seen that psychiatric research can be value-laden and that this value-ladenness can have pernicious effects. Now we must ask how things might be made better.

8.4.1 Suggestion 1: make science value-free

The discussion above should have made it clear that making science value-free is a non-starter. To give just some examples of the ways in which science is necessarily value laden, scientific research has to be directed at particular areas, background assumptions have to be used in making sense of raw data, and the testimony of some witnesses must be rejected as untrustworthy.

8.4.2 Suggestion 2: be aware of our values

Sometimes it is suggested that researchers can overcome the problems caused by value-ladenness if they strive to be aware of their values when they conduct research. This suggestion is probably most commonly found in guides to methodology in the social sciences. To take an example, Philip Banyard writes: "Balance and objectivity is not possible. What is important is to be aware of your perspective and the limitations it imposes on your view" (1999: 78). The basic problem with this idea is that very often people are not aware of the influence of their own values. In the papers I have studied it is clear that many researchers implicitly assumed that the best people were people like them. But no one would ever explicitly think "Middle-class white men from my home town are best and I conduct my research on this basis". When our own reasoning is shaped by our values this is hard to spot because we will tend to perceive our reasoning as being justified by the nature of reality. So, to modern eyes some of the researchers discussed in the previous section were clearly biased against people from certain ethnic groups. However, I suggest that the researchers themselves would not have seen things this way. Instead, they thought that their research findings reflected the nature of the world. So, when O'Malley writes that coloured people are at an earlier evolutionary stage, we can see this belief as motivated by the assumption that black people are of lesser worth than white people. O'Malley, however, would presumably have thought that she held such beliefs simply because she considered them to be true.

To take a more recent example, consider the assumption that people with learning disabilities cannot conduct academic research. A decade or so ago this assumption was almost universally accepted as being true. It was not thought to reflect any bias against people with learning disabilities; instead it was simply taken to be a natural fact that people with learning disabilities lack academic ability. More recently, however, this assumption has been challenged. People with learning disabilities are now engaged in producing research.[3]

What these examples show is that value-laden assumptions are hard to spot when the values are our own. Stephen Jay Gould (1981) reaches a similar conclusion in his study of the history of intelligence testing. Gould notes that much of the work he studied was clearly shaped by sexist and racist assumptions. Still he concludes, "few conscious ideologues have entered these debates on either side. Scientists needn't become explicit apologists for their class or culture in order to reflect these pervasive aspects of life" (*ibid.*: 21).

8.4.3 Suggestion 3: make sure the research is laden with "good" values

Some researchers have proposed doing emancipatory research (Stone & Priestley 1996). Here the idea is that the problems of value-ladenness can be overcome by loading research with good values. However, one fundamental problem with seeking to produce "emancipatory" research is that it is often unclear which theories or hypotheses are the truly emancipatory ones. For example, different gay activists have reacted very differently to the idea that homosexuality might have some genetic basis (Koertge 2000: §54). Some have held that it is good to think that homosexuality is genetically based: that way homosexuals cannot be held to blame for their orientation. Others have seen the search for genes linked to homosexuality as linked to efforts to pathologize homosexuality. Similarly, feminists are split on the question of whether it is better to see women as being fundamentally like or unlike men.

8.4.4 Suggestion 4: have the right kinds of people do research

The idea that the problems of value-ladenness can be reduced if only the right kinds of people do research comes in two strengths: strong and modest. Here I shall consider each claim in turn.

Strong standpoint epistemology

On the strong version, problems of value-ladenness can be overcome if research into oppressed groups is conducted by the members of those groups. Such claims have been put forward by a variety of people, including some feminists, some disability activists and some Deaf researchers. These thinkers have claimed, respectively, that research into women should be done by women, research on disabled people should be done by disabled people, and research into Deaf people should be done by Deaf people. Consider the following claim by Paddy Ladd *et al.*:

> Research affecting Deaf people and their lives must be Deaf-led; originating with Deaf people, coordinated by Deaf people and disseminated by Deaf people for the empowerment of the Deaf community. Any other level of involvement, especially within an academy whose stated aim is the attainment of "full knowledge" simply renders the research invalid. (2003: 27)

To my knowledge, so far no one has claimed that research into mental illness should be *controlled* by mentally ill people, although an increasing number of authors argue that service-users should have greater involvement in the research process (Thornicroft *et al.* 2002; Townend & Braithwaite 2002; Trivedi & Wykes 2002; Telford & Faulkner 2004; Thomas and Bracken 2004; Glasby & Beresford 2006). However, given the ways in which the claims of the user movement tend to follow those made by disability rights activists, it will probably only be a matter of time before claims are made that research into mental illness should be controlled by the mentally ill.

Sometimes the claim that research on some oppressed group should be conducted exclusively by members of that group is argued for on political grounds. Here the thought is that knowledge is power, and so for a group to claim the right to study themselves is empowering. I will not deal with such claims here. Here I am concerned only with the idea that research conducted by members of an oppressed group is epistemically superior.

The idea that certain oppressed groups are in an epistemically privileged position is derived from Marxist theory (Lukács [1923] 1971). Here the idea is that the proletariat are epistemically privileged. They are epistemically privileged because their oppression is what makes the social system work. As such, in noticing their oppression, members of the proletariat can potentially gain insight into the workings of the social system as a whole. This idea has been extended by some feminists who argue that the reproductive labour of women is central to the functioning of patriarchal capitalist societies (e.g. Rose 1987). The plausibility of these claims can be disputed. But one thing that should be noticed is that it is hard to see how such positions can be extended to groups such as disabled people, Deaf people, or mental health service users. It is true that these groups have been and are oppressed. It may also be true that capitalist societies are particularly likely to oppress such people; so, for example, Foucault (1971) suggests that the mentally ill came to be perceived as a group in part because they cannot be made to work. Still, it is not plausible that the oppression of disabled people, or Deaf people, or mentally ill people, is *central* to the workings of capitalist society. I conclude that full-blooded Marxist or feminist versions of standpoint epistemology cannot be straightforwardly extended to the case of disabled people or Deaf people or mental health service users.

Moving away from the full theory of Marxist versions of standpoint epistemology, some have suggested that those who are oppressed are more likely to gain insight into their oppression because they have no interests in obscuring it. However, it is not always true that those who are unfortunate are the most able to perceive the true causes of their misfortune. Consider the following two cases. First, suppose a student gains poor marks for his essays and that this is because they are not very good. The student forms the belief that the lecturer dislikes him and has marked him down. Now, of course, on occasion lecturers do hand out poor marks to those they dislike. However, while such occurrences are unusual, it is quite common for students to believe that they have been unfairly given low marks. Such examples show that under some circumstances the unfortunate have a tendency to attribute their misfortune to oppression when they are not actually oppressed. Conversely, consider a case where a student *is* given low marks because a lecturer dislikes him. In many such cases the fact that this has occurred will be more easily known by the lecturer than by the student (the lecturer may be able to remember intentionally deducting marks, for example). These examples show that whether the truth about some matter is most easily accessible to the oppressed or the oppressor depends on the details of the situation. There is no general link between being oppressed and being in an epistemically privileged position.

Modest standpoint epistemology

Modest standpoint epistemology does not claim that one particular group should have exclusive rights to investigate some particular domain. Rather, it claims that particular sources of information may be differentially available to different kinds of investigator. So, people who live in Lancaster are more likely than those who live in Bristol to know which Lancaster pubs are the best; people with eczema are more likely to know whether eczema hurts than those without eczema, and so on.

In support of modest standpoint epistemology we can consider Rutherford Stevens's 1947 paper "Racial Aspects of Emotional Problems of Negro Soldiers". Rutherford, who was himself a black psychiatrist, notes that he had certain advantages over his white colleagues. He writes that it was especially difficult for white medical officers to understand black soldiers because "most of them have been subjected throughout their life to many false concepts of the Negro" (1947: 493). He goes on to note that white psychiatrists frequently misinterpret the personal histories of black soldiers: "Certainly many fail to understand that a history of intermittent school attendance and frequent changes of jobs is not in some communities indicative of emotional instability, but the result of an effort to survive" (*ibid*.: 497). Although Stevens himself does not mention the possibility, other writers have suggested that black patients might be happy to tell black psychiatrists things that they would not tell white medics (Fernando 2002: 105). It is plausible that, as he had different background knowledge, and different access to the subject population, certain truths were more accessible to Stevens than to his white colleagues.

To move to a current example, consider recent calls within psychiatry to increase the influence of researchers from poor countries (Saxena *et al*. 2003; Tyrer 2005). Researchers from rich countries currently dominate the editorial boards of medical journals and write the vast majority of published papers. One reason why this is problematic is that certain truths will be more accessible to researchers from poor countries (most obviously such researchers will have greater access to facts about the psychological consequences of poverty). As such, if such researchers do not get to play a full role in the scientific community the community as a whole loses out.

For the modest standpoint epistemologist, researchers from different backgrounds are not interchangeable. Depending on the question at issue, some will be in a better position to discover the answer than others. Different people have access to different facts, and their different interests make it likely that they will notice different things. As such, it is better to have a greater variety of researchers engaged in an area of research. That way the chances of truths being accessible to at least one researcher are increased.

8.4.5 Suggestion 5: scientists can correct each others' shortcomings

Of the various types of value-ladenness that I have discussed some can be viewed as being "internal" to the scientific process (i.e. it is the scientists' values that count) while others are "external" (i.e. they involve the values of funders/politicians and so on). This division is only rough, as the status of some concerns will be unclear (what about the interests of scientists who sit on funding councils, for example?). Still, the distinction will serve for our purposes.

My study has focused on value-ladenness as displayed in articles in the *American Journal of Psychiatry* concerning race between 1844 and 1962. As such, I am only in a position to discuss how problems of value-ladenness that are "internal" to the scientific process can be dealt with. The debates in the *American Journal of Psychiatry* give us reason for optimism. I suggest that when evaluating the effects of value-ladenness we should focus on research programmes, rather than on individual papers. This is because the general consensus that is reached on a question is generally more influential than the views of any one author. Looking through the debates in the *American Journal of Psychiatry*, we can see that the biases of individual papers can often be corrected by authors with different viewpoints. This point is missed by studies on value-ladenness that focus on individual papers. In so far as such studies selectively pick out examples of perniciously value-laden papers they present the problems of value-ladenness as being worse than they really are.[4]

It is worth noting how the debates about race in the *American Journal of Psychiatry* that we have looked at were eventually resolved. In the end it came to be generally accepted that, compared to slaves, free coloured people do not suffer from excessive mental illness; that Italians, Jews and Slavs do not suffer from excessive rates of mental illness; and that the causes of high rates of mental illness among black people are more likely to be sociological (racism, hospital provision, etc.) than due to natural biological differences. I suggest that it was easier for scientists with certain values to reach these conclusions, but that eventually these conclusions became generally accepted because they were better supported by the data (in so far as the background assumptions that had to be made to get from the data to the conclusions were more plausible). For example, focusing on the debate over the interpretation of high rates of hospital admission among the foreign-born population of New York, it was easier for scientists who expected there to be no difference in the rates to see that an adjustment needed to be made because of the age distribution of the populations. However, once the arguments for this adjustment had been made they could be seen to be reasonable and accepted by everybody.

Here I do not mean to urge complacency. My view is not that everything will always work out okay in the end. Obviously when we look back at the history of science we can see that value-ladenness can cause problems that persist for considerable lengths of time. Still there is some reason for optimism when we bear in mind that:

- science is a social process – it is the research programme rather than individual papers that matters;
- researchers with different viewpoints can spot problems that others overlook; and
- once a researcher has spotted a problem others can appreciate their arguments regardless of their initial outlook.

This suggests that to minimize the problems caused by value-ladenness we should seek (i) a diverse body of researchers, and (ii) a system in which debate is encouraged (e.g. one where it is easy for those who spot problems with a paper to publish their objections). These conclusions are very similar to those argued for by Helen Longino in *Science as Social Knowledge* (1990) and, looking further back, to those reached by Ernst Nagel in 1961. As Nagel puts it:

> the difficulties generated for scientific inquiry by unconscious bias and tacit value orientations … are usually overcome, often only gradually, through the self-corrective mechanisms of science as a social enterprise. For modern science encourages the invention, the mutual exchange, and the free but responsible criticism of ideas; it welcomes competition in the quest for knowledge between independent investigators, even where their intellectual orientations are different; and it progressively diminishes the effects of bias by retaining only those proposed conclusions of its inquiries that survive critical examination by an indefinitely large community of students, whatever their value preferences or doctrinal commitments. (1961: 489–90)

This chapter adds somewhat to Longino's and Nagel's claims in so far as here the conclusions are argued for semi-empirically, by looking at how the problems of value-ladenness have played out in actual debates, whereas Longino and Nagel argue for their positions on *a priori* grounds.

At this point two caveats should be noted. First, the suggestion that scientists can correct each other's biases only helps with value-ladenness that is internal to the scientific process. The values of the funders of research can still have a pernicious influence and as yet I have no suggestion as to how such problems might be dealt with. Secondly, the papers in the *American Journal of Psychiatry* that I have looked at involve fairly simple debates. It was easy for individual researchers to find problems with the studies and publish their disagreements. It might be harder to correct the effect of biases in "big science" undertaken by teams of researchers. When the reasoning involved in a study is more complicated and also distributed among different researchers, problems might be harder to spot. (On the other hand research that is undertaken by teams may involve a greater number of viewpoints to begin with).

8.5 Conclusion

To summarize, in this chapter I have argued that psychiatric research is value-laden at every stage and that value-ladenness can be epistemically pernicious. Plausibly, psychiatry is not special in this respect. Other sciences are value-laden too. However, I have suggested that the problems caused by value-ladenness can be minimized. It is important to remember that science is a social process, and that it is generally the research programme rather than individual papers that matters. We can thus limit the effects of value-ladenness by promoting a diverse body of researchers who are able to criticize each other. Researchers with different viewpoints will be able to spot problems that others overlook, and once a researcher has spotted a problem others can appreciate their arguments regardless of their initial outlook.

9. Managing values and interests 2
Big business and judging treatments

Much psychiatric research is paid for, monitored and publicized by the pharmaceutical industry. Pharmaceutical companies need to make money, and when this goal conflicts with discovering the truth about mental illness they cannot afford to care too much about truth. The problems caused by this are well documented, and we shall see how financial considerations have led to a distortion of psychiatric theory. In this chapter I focus particularly on the use of randomized controlled trials (RCTs) to assess treatment efficacy. Multiple difficult decisions have to be made when designing an RCT, and it is possible for interested parties to make these decisions with an eye to obtaining particular results. This means that industry-sponsored trials can frequently obtain the results they desire.

In the past few years, many writers have discussed the ways in which psychiatric research has been distorted by the pharmaceutical industry (e.g. Healy 1997; 2002; Angell 2005; Safer 2002), and this has resulted in a crisis of confidence in efficacy studies. The running of clinical trials has long been heavily regulated. Nevertheless, in the past few years various new mechanisms have been introduced or proposed in attempts to further control the practices of researchers and to ensure the trustworthiness of psychiatric research. In the second part of the chapter, I diagnose what has gone wrong with the use of RCTs in psychiatry. I use ideas from Steven Shapin and Simon Schaffer's *Leviathan and the Air-Pump* (1985) to argue that for any area of science to be trustworthy it is necessary for mechanisms for policing testimony to be in place. In recent years, these mechanisms have broken down within psychiatry, and proposed new regulations and practices seek to shore them up.

I finish by arguing that the case of RCTs in psychiatry shows that traditional epistemology and philosophy of science have taken too narrow a focus when thinking about scientific method. These fields have assumed that the seekers of knowledge are disinterested. But they are not. Thus, as well as considering how ideal knowledge-seekers might proceed, we need to consider how non-ideal, socially situated actors can be constrained to discover and share truths. Taking such a perspective leads one to view methodologies, such as the use of RCTs, differently. While a well-designed RCT may be the perfect way for an ideal knowledge-seeker to gain data on effectiveness, the use of RCTs by less than ideal data-seekers may be problematic.

9.1 An introduction to randomized controlled trials

Working out whether a new treatment is better than an existing treatment is frequently difficult: individual variations among human beings mean that even the best treatment will probably not work for everybody. Conversely, some patients will get better even if they are given no drugs at all. Differences between two treatments may also be slight. This means that it is not generally possible for individual patients or doctors to evaluate whether a treatment is effective merely by trying it out. Competing drugs will need to be given to large subject populations, and statistical techniques employed, to determine whether one drug really does bring about improvements over another.

Furthermore, when drugs are given to test populations, it is important to be sure that the two populations are similar in relevant respects. Suppose, for example, that a new and expensive drug just goes to those who can afford it. This group may then do better. Here, though, the test of the drug would be unfair, as there is a chance that the rich improved for a reason unconnected to their drug use, for example, because they could buy better food. For the test to be fair the populations who take the test drug and those who do not have to be relevantly alike. In addition, the placebo effect causes problems. The placebo effect means that patients have a tendency to get better when they expect to get better. New and impressive-looking pills can thus bring benefits regardless of their active ingredients.

RCTs are designed to get around all these problems. Let us take for illustration a case where two drugs are under test. Members of the subject population are allocated randomly to one of two groups. Randomization ensures that the two groups can be expected to be alike with respect to both known and unknown variables (whether this has been achieved can be monitored by checking that the members of the two groups do not differ in respects that are known to be significant). One group of subjects then gets one drug. The other group gets the other. In a double-blind trial neither the subjects nor the administering physicians know who is getting which drug. All the subjects are monitored for measures of improvement. Statistical techniques are then used to see whether one group does significantly better than the other.

RCTs have long been considered the gold standard for assessing the efficacy of psychoactive medications. The US FDA has required RCT-based evidence that drugs are effective since 1962, and more recently RCTs have received an additional boost through the broad acceptance of the evidence based medicine movement.

There has been a great deal of discussion of the methodological and ethical problems associated with the use of RCTs: many authors have worried that an emphasis on RCTs has led to other types of evidence – such as the individual case study – being undervalued (Williams & Garner 2002). Richard Ashcroft (2004) argues that RCT methodology implicitly commits one to various assumptions about the nature of probability judgements. Discussion of the ethics of RCTs have focused on the deception that RCTs often require, or on worries that half the patients in the trial will of necessity receive sub-optimal treatment.[1] All of these discussions are important, but here we shall restrict our attention to just three potential difficulties with the use of RCTs. These will serve to show that difficult decisions have to be made when designing RCTs and that evaluating treatments can often be problematic. We shall see (i) that RCTs can only be as good as the methods used to select subject populations, (ii) that RCTs can only be as good as the methods used to judge success and (iii) that RCTs are better suited to judging certain types of treatment than others.

9.2 Problems with evaluating the effectiveness of treatments

9.2.1 Problems with selecting subject populations and generalizing results

The results of an RCT will only be generalizable if the subject population has been selected in the right way. Nowadays most clinical trials select subject populations on the basis of diagnosis. Diagnostic criteria, such as those provided by the DSM, are used to pick out patients suffering from, say, a major depressive episode. The results of the trial are then thought to be applicable to patients with the same diagnosis in clinical settings. The reasoning involved here assumes that the disorders of all people who conform to the criteria for a major depressive episode are fundamentally similar. Maybe, for example, all cases are caused by a particular imbalance in neurotransmitters that the drugs help rectify. But, regardless of the precise similarity, the cases are assumed to be fundamentally alike; this is why they can all be expected to respond in the same way.

Most RCTs select subject populations on the basis of diagnosis, and for the results of such trials to be generalizable, such diagnostic categories have to validly reflect the nature of mental disorders. Many authors, however, doubt the validity of current diagnostic categories and for this reason are dubious of the validity of clinical trials in mental health. So, for example, John Marzillier worries that "The whole business of categorising people's problems into quasi-medical and suspect diagnoses is psychologically dubious, and outcome studies in psychotherapy tell clinicians nothing of value" (2004: 393–4).

I argued in Chapter 4 that at least some types of mental disorder can reasonably be considered natural kinds. As a consequence, I think that in principle there is nothing problematic about generalizing from RCTs where subject populations are selected on the basis of diagnosis (providing, of course, that the diagnostic criteria in use do indeed succeed in picking out a natural kind of disorder). Here, however, I wish to respond in another way to those who doubt the reliability of RCTs because they doubt that mental disorders fall into kinds. At present most RCTs select subject populations on the basis of diagnosis, but as I shall show this does not need to be the case. RCTs can be employed whenever the subject populations and those the results will be applied to are alike in the respects that are relevant to the action of the drug under test. Depending on how we think a particular drug works, different methods of selecting subject populations will thus be appropriate. Here I shall make this point clearer by considering three different models of drug action. These models are not intended to be exhaustive, but are simply aimed at showing that we can think of drugs as working in a variety of different ways.

- *Model 1: The "chemical straitjacket" model.* Straitjackets do not cure or reduce symptoms (a person with schizophrenia who is restrained still has schizophrenia and still hears voices) but they do make patients easier to manage. The "chemical straitjacket" model of drug action claims that psychoactive drugs act like straitjackets: they block socially problematic behaviours but do not do much else. A pure example of a chemical straitjacket drug would be a drug that controls behaviour by putting patients to sleep or by stopping them moving. The problematic behaviour is prevented, but the patient's disorder remains the same. It is worth noting that chemical straitjacket drugs will act in a similar way on anyone who takes them. When one takes a chemical straitjacket drug it does not matter whether one suffers from depression, or schizophrenia, or nothing at all: the drug will prevent certain behaviours in anyone who takes it.
- *Model 2: The "target symptom" model.* Painkillers are examples of drugs that target symptoms. Drugs that fit the "target symptom" model act on specific symptoms regardless of their cause. As such, when taking painkillers, whether one's headache is caused by a hangover, flu or head injury does not matter: the painkiller will reduce the pain whatever its cause. Unlike chemical straitjacket drugs, drugs that fit the target symptom model do not do anything much if they are taken by people who do not have the symptom that the drug acts on. Painkillers stop pain, but if one is not in pain then little happens.

- *Model 3: The "magic bullet" model.* Drugs that fit the "magic bullet" model attack the cause of a disorder. Antibiotics are good examples of drugs that fit the magic bullet model. Various diseases are caused by bacteria. Antibiotics kill the bacteria, and so cure the disease. When using a magic bullet drug, accurate diagnosis is important, as different magic bullets will work for different disorders.

  One clear indication that someone implicitly adopts a magic bullet model of drug action is that they take data regarding treatment effectiveness to be a valuable resource for determining how mental disorders should be classified. For example, theorists have argued that anxiety with panic attacks should be picked out from other types of anxiety on the basis of its response to Imipramine (Klein & Fink 1962), and that when patient populations respond similarly to antidepressants this means that their conditions should be grouped together (Hudson & Pope 1990). Such attempts at the "psychopharmacological dissection" of disorders implicitly rely on the idea that drugs treat specific disorders, and this assumption is characteristic of the magic bullet model.

Some writers have claimed that one or other of these models fits all drugs. Elsewhere I have argued that such claims have often been motivated by guild interests (the interests of analysts have been served by target symptom models, while magic bullet models suit biologically oriented psychiatrists better) (Cooper 2005: ch. 4).[2] I think that those who claim that all drugs accord with one model are wrong and that it is plausible that different drugs work in different ways. In some cases a drug's action may best be conceptualized using a chemical straitjacket model, while other drugs better fit a target symptom model or magic bullet model. Often it will be possible to discover empirically which model best fits the action of a particular drug: chemical straitjacket drugs have effects on everyone; target symptom drugs affect a particular symptom whatever its cause; magic bullet drugs only work on a particular diagnosis.

Depending on the model of drug action that one adopts, different methods of selecting the subject population for an RCT will seem appropriate. A chemical straitjacket drug acts on everyone in the same way. In testing such drugs the subject populations merely need to be made up of human beings. A target symptom drug acts on particular symptoms. In testing such drugs, subject populations will be selected on the basis of symptoms. Magic bullet drugs act on particular disease processes. In testing these drugs, subject populations need to be selected on the basis of diagnosis.

Much current psychiatric literature assumes a magic bullet model of drug action, although prior to the 1970s other models were more popular (*ibid.*). Still, it is possible to design trials that do not rely on diagnosis to select subject populations. Consider Eisenberg and Rozan (1960), who used a target symptom model to investigate the mood-elevating effects of chlorphenoxamine HCl. All their subjects suffered from depressed mood, although they had diverse diagnoses including neurotic depression, undifferentiated schizophrenia and organic brain disorders. Indeed, as late as 1970, a textbook advised researchers to select subject groups on the basis of symptoms as "Patients with the same diagnosis may be quite heterogeneous, and their symptoms and their disabling features may require different therapy" (Okun 1970: 386).

In Chapter 4 I argued that at least some mental disorders are likely to be natural kinds. I thus think that there is nothing intrinsically problematic about RCTs that select subject populations on the basis of diagnosis. The point of this section has been to argue that those who disagree with me about mental disorders being natural kinds can still use RCTs. For an RCT to make sense it just needs to be the case that the subject population is relevantly like the populations that will be treated: depending on the particular drug, simply being human or sharing the same symptoms may be enough for this condition to be met.

It is not necessary to select a subject population on the basis of diagnosis. However, most current drug trials do in fact use diagnosis to pick out subject groups. When RCTs are designed in this manner, a question arises about the fineness of diagnostic splitting that is appropriate. Most psychiatric diagnoses fall into families of related disorders. So schizophrenia falls within the psychotic disorders, for example, and schizophrenia itself can be split into numerous subtypes. A trial might choose to select a subject population who have all been diagnosed as suffering from a psychotic disorder, or who all have schizophrenia, or who all have catatonic schizophrenia. Depending on how one thinks the drug works (is it thought to affect a pathological mechanism that is common to all psychotic disorders or specific to catatonic schizophrenia?) different decisions here will make more or less sense. The decision about how finely to cut diagnoses in a trial is very important, as trials that select different subject groups may well produce different findings. Parallel problems will also affect RCTs that choose subject populations on the basis of a target symptom. Here too decisions will need to be made about how similar symptoms need to be before they are grouped together.

Once the subject population has been chosen, worries may still arise as to how similar the subject population is to the population that will eventually receive the drug treatment. A distinction may be drawn between a drug being of proven "efficacy", that is, working in an RCT, and being of proven "effectiveness", that is, working in the clinic (see e.g. Schoenwald & Hoagwood 2001). Most RCTs exclude many potential subjects. Commonly, for example, they leave out those who suffer from co-morbid conditions, old people and pregnant women. Still, the results drawn from the RCT are then used to guide treatment decisions relating to a more diverse population. This can throw the applicability of the results of trials into doubt.

Malcolm Parker (2005) has argued that at least concerns about co-morbidity can be minimized. Parker thinks that the results of trials can be applied to patients with co-morbid conditions even when such patients are excluded from trials. When patients suffer from co-morbid conditions, Parker thinks a particular disorder can still be abstracted away from the rest and be treated in accordance with trial results. To illustrate, if a patient suffers from depression, antidepressants can be used to treat this aspect of their condition regardless of the fact that they also suffer from a learning disability. However, Parker accepts that applying results in cases where the various conditions of a patient are causally related may be more problematic. And, unfortunately, in psychiatry, the various conditions that a patient suffers from are likely to causally interact in complex ways. For example, if I suffer from alcoholism and schizophrenia then I am likely to skip doses of antipsychotics so I can go drinking and this may make my schizophrenia harder to treat. Similarly, if I am depressed and also a psychopath then my belief that everyone hates me may not be amenable to correction with cognitive therapy, because it may be true. Where conditions interact, applying the results of RCTs may be difficult.

To summarize, for the results of an RCT to be generalizable, the subject population needs to be relevantly similar to the population that will be treated with the drug. This condition can be met even if there is reason to be sceptical of the idea that clearly demarcated disorders can be distinguished, because, for example, trials that compare groups of people with similar symptoms might be used instead. In cases where the population tested is different from that treated in relevant ways (e.g. with respect to causally interacting co-morbid conditions) there may well be problems with generalizing from the results of a clinical trial. Selecting suitable subject populations for an RCT is thus far from straightforward. As a consequence determining whether a treatment is effective can be difficult.

9.2.2 Problems with determining success

In an RCT, groups of patients are given different treatments and then their progress is monitored. The point of the trial is to see which group does better, and frequently batteries of assessment scales will be used to assess the treatment outcomes.

Often deciding what sorts of outcomes should be looked for is difficult. A mentally ill person may suffer from a wide range of symptoms and drugs often produce a range of effects. Deciding which effects are most significant and which are desirable may not be easy. Take the case of someone who hears voices and gets distressed by this. Suppose that with one drug treatment they continue to hear voices but are now able to ignore them, while a different drug stops the voices all together. How are the outcomes of these treatments to be compared?

Are voices only a problem if they cause distress? Or should treatment aim to silence even harmless voices? Once one takes into account that the two drugs will almost certainly also produce a different range of side effects the judgement as to which is best becomes even harder.

In some cases even determining whether a drug effect should be classed as "successful symptom reduction" or "side effect" can be awkward. For example, many of those who take medications for bipolar disorder or attention-deficit/hyperactivity disorder (ADHD) find that the drugs dampen their emotional responses. To a certain extent this is how these drugs work. However, the ambiguity of the effects is nicely captured in this description of the effects of lithium on patients who are hypomanic: "It is as if their 'intensity of living' dial had been turned down a few notches. Things do not seem so very important, or imperative; there is a greater acceptance of everyday life as it is rather than as one might want it to be" (Dyson & Mendelson 1968: 545, cited in Breggin 1993: 219). Nothing has gone wrong when lithium "turns down the intensity of living dial": this is what the drug is supposed to do. But the value of this action is ambiguous.

Those with different theoretical outlooks may also judge the severity of different symptoms differently and hope for different things from a good treatment. To take an example, therapists from a psychodynamic orientation have traditionally placed great weight on whether a patient gains insight into their condition (so, roughly, on whether the patient comes to accept they have a problem, and that it is rooted in psychological conflict). In contrast, therapists from other traditions, and patients themselves, frequently consider insight to be relatively unimportant (Dimsdale *et al.* 1979). Depending on whether one considers insight to matter, different treatments will seem effective.[3]

When theorists have different views as to what counts as a symptom, they will disagree over the effectiveness of treatments. Furthermore there may be disagreements as to whether symptom reduction should even be the primary goal of treatment. As an alternative, some suggest that the aim of treatment is to improve a patient's quality of life. Especially in cases where a drug reduces symptoms, but has side effects or is awkward to take, those who seek to improve quality of life and those who seek symptom reduction will view the treatment very differently. For example, consider the weight that should be placed on the fact that patients cannot drink alcohol while taking some psychoactive drugs. Some people with schizophrenia will skip medication so they can drink (e.g. Knowles 2000: 130). Medics tend to have been trained to view symptom-reduction as the end of treatment, and are thus disposed to view such behaviour unfavourably, as medication needs to be taken regularly for maximum effectiveness. However, in the alcohol-fuelled culture of the UK, for someone to be unable to drink for a long period of time can be a very real evil. At least in certain communities, the teetotal tend to be excluded from the activities of their peers. Thus while the drugs may help to control symptoms, in preventing someone from drinking they can reduce that person's quality of life.

Similarly, different parties differ in the importance that they attach to side effects. In general, health professionals place more value on symptom reduction, while patients worry more about side effects (Lenert *et al.* 2000). Again, depending on the importance granted to side effects, the degree to which a particular drug is judged a success will vary.

Parker (2005: 27–8) suggests that these difficulties with judging drug effects can be overcome to a substantial extent. He suggests that guidelines can be expressed as hypothetical imperatives. Instead of simply saying "Drug *x* is effective for schizophrenia", guidelines should say things such as "If you want to stop voices and do not mind a 10 per cent risk of concentration problems take drug *y*" and "If you do not mind the voices staying as long as they do not upset you anymore take drug *z*". In an ideal world Parker's suggestion would be useful, but in one where there are substantial pressures for drugs to be ranked in terms of cost-effectiveness they may be hard to put into practice.

Groups can disagree as to what counts as a symptom, disagree as to whether a treatment effect is desirable, and disagree as to whether the end of treatment is symptom reduction or improving a patient's quality of life. In addition, it is worth noting that drug treatments are sometimes given with the primary aim of benefiting other people rather than the patient. Considering whether the use of drugs to control socially awkward behaviour is justifiable is beyond the scope of this book. Here I just note that it happens,[4] and that groups who use drugs with the aim of controlling problematic behaviour will have different views as to which drugs are most effective.

Depending on what one wants a drug to do, different drugs will seem effective. In general, patients are keen to use drugs to improve their quality of life, while other people are keen to use drugs to reduce symptoms or to control problematic behaviour. To date, health professionals have written the ratings scales for assessing drug outcomes and so their views have tended to carry more weight, but recently there have been calls for users' views on treatment to be granted more importance (Perkins 2001; Hellewell 2002). If users do gain the power to judge drugs, one can expect that views as to which drugs are effective will change. We can conclude that working out whether a drug is effective is frequently problematic because it is frequently hard to decide exactly what we want drug use to achieve.

9.2.3 Randomized controlled trials are better suited for judging certain types of treatment

RCTs work best for evaluating treatments that can be placebo controlled, that are employed over a short amount of time, and where the effects produced can be measured in quantitative terms. When treatments cannot adequately meet these requirements they will be disadvantaged in a system that takes RCTs to be the gold standard for assessing effectiveness. Here we shall examine the problems faced by attempts to use RCTs to test psychotherapies as an example.

Psychoactive medications have long been assessed via RCTs, in large part because such evidence is required before most countries will approve use of a drug. In the absence of such regulatory pressures, the use of clinical trials for assessing psychotherapies has lagged behind. However, the funders of care are increasingly unwilling to pay for treatments until they have been proved effective, and so pressure to conduct trials in psychotherapy is mounting (Parry 2000).

However, running RCTs to assess psychotherapies is particularly difficult. In an RCT to test a drug half the subjects can be given a placebo, and the trial can be blinded so that neither the subjects nor the clinicians know which drug each subject receives. In a trial of psychotherapies, on the other hand, it is not clear what the equivalent of a drug placebo would be. Some trials have compared a specific therapy with mere clinical management, but even in the case of clinical management a relationship builds up between the doctor and patient, and some therapists claim that this in itself could be expected to be therapeutic. In addition, neither patients nor therapists can be blind regarding the nature of the treatment that the patient receives: if a course of behavioural therapy is undertaken this will be obvious to both patient and therapist (*ibid.*).

There are also problems with standardizing the nature of the therapy that patients receive. A pill will contain a standard dose of standard ingredients, but the therapy provided by different therapists can vary substantially. As Marzillier puts it, "Like friendship, romance or chatting to someone in your local shop, psychotherapy is at heart a personal transaction … How can such complexity be reduced to a set of predetermined treatments …?" (2004: 394).

In general, trials have attempted to get round this problem by training therapists with treatment manuals (Chambless & Ollendick 2001). The manual sets out the principles and procedures of the particular therapy under test, and gives examples of what the therapist should do in particular circumstances. At least to a certain extent, it can be hoped that the use of such manuals will ensure that the therapy provided by different therapists is the same. In addition, in cases where one therapist treats a good number of patients, statistical techniques can be used to compare the efficacy of different individual therapists.

A further problem with using trials to judge the efficacy of different forms of psychotherapy is that different psychotherapies can be expected to work over different timescales. Even the adherents of psychodynamic treatments only expect to see patients improve over a longish duration, while a much shorter course of treatment might be appropriate for cognitive or behavioural therapies. Nevertheless, clinical trials by their very nature tend to be run over periods of weeks or months rather than years. Longer trials are seldom performed because drop-out rates tend to reach unacceptable levels. This means that outcomes research in psychotherapy has a built in tendency to favour certain therapies over others.

Despite these difficulties, evidence-based approaches are increasingly applied to psychotherapies,[5] and this trend will doubtless continue. Outcomes research in mental health is here to stay, and when the results are intelligently interpreted it is surely a good thing. However, as we have seen, problems with selecting subject populations, problems with rating success and the special problems with assessing psychotherapies together mean that determining whether a particular treatment works is a far from straightforward matter.

9.3 Social epistemology and the breakdown of trust in psychiatry

In designing an RCT, multiple and potentially problematic decisions have to be taken. Among other decisions, researchers have to make decisions regarding:

- the subject group;
- the outcomes that are to be monitored;
- the timescale;
- whether the treatment will be compared with another treatment or placebo; and
- the doses of the treatments to be used.

In addition, it should be remembered that RCTs are often necessarily large and expensive studies that are thus hard to replicate. In this section I suggest that the intrinsic difficulties with running an RCT have made them vulnerable to manipulation by those with interests in the production of specific results, most notably drug companies. There is currently a crisis concerning the credibility of psychiatric research and I argue that this is linked in part to the use of RCTs.

Pharmaceutical companies fund most research into drug therapies in psychiatry. A recent sample suggests that around 60 per cent of drug trials are industry funded (Perlis *et al.* 2005). When clinical trials are funded by pharmaceutical companies, the results that are eventually reported have been found to differ significantly from independent studies. Roy Perlis *et al.* examined a sample of clinical trials published between 2001 and 2003. They found that those that reported conflict of interest were 4.9 times more likely to record positive results for the drug under study. C. Bruce Baker *et al.* (2003) similarly found that studies sponsored by selective serotonin reuptake inhibitor (**SSRI**) manufacturers were more likely to find use of their drugs to be cost-effective than non-industry-sponsored studies.

Industry-funded investigators are more likely to obtain positive results, but it is not clear whether this is *because* they are industry-funded. An alternative explanation may be that clinicians tend to agree to industry collaboration only when they believe that the product under test is a good one (Lakoff 2005: 149). Conceivably, these physicians are then more likely to find positive results because of their positive expectations rather than because of financial incentives. But in any event, there is a correlation between a study being industry funded and it finding positive results, and this is sufficient to throw doubt on the credibility of such studies.

As a consequence, a numbers of commentators have noted that psychiatric research is now in crisis. David Healy notes that "the evidence that practice is supposed to follow is losing its credibility" (2002: 312). Gilbody and Song worry that "in many areas publication might be seen as a sophisticated marketing tool by the sponsors of research" (2000: 255). As we shall see, a number of factors act together to enable pharmaceutical companies to shape the results that are reported.

9.3.1 Getting the right results

The design of clinical trials is heavily regulated, and readers should not get the impression that drug companies can run trials however they like. Protocols and data sets get checked at numerous points by a complex array of regulatory bodies, "monitors" and independent auditors; see the rules set out in International Conference on Harmonisation of Technical Requirements for Registration of Pharmaceuticals for Human Use (ICH) (1996), for example. Occasionally, perhaps, investigators "lose" patients down the back of a filing cabinet, or make "copying errors" when transferring outcomes data, but procedures are in place that aim to catch such malpractice. Nevertheless, even if outright fraud is unusual, a company that needs to obtain particular results from a trial has ways of ensuring that it obtains those results.

As we saw in the previous section, numerous difficult decisions have to be made about trial design. When it comes to picking subject populations, or the criteria for judging success, multiple possible choices might be justifiable. It is often possible to make these decisions in such a way that a result that is favourable to the company's drug is more likely. Furthermore, as these choices *are* complex and contested, it is hard for those who make particular interested decisions to be challenged.

Currently, the sample populations for an RCT are almost always selected on the basis of diagnosis. This means that whether a drug will be found to be effective depends in part on whether clusters of disorders are lumped together or split apart. A drug that is not effective for a cluster of disorders may still be effective for some more specific condition. In such cases a company that wants to show that the drug is effective can select to test it on a narrow type, while a company that wants to hide its effectiveness can test it on the broader group. In *The Antidepressant Era*, Healy discusses the case of clomipramine and obsessive compulsive disorder (1997: 199–208). Geigy, manufacturers of clomipramine, had originally intended to market it as a general antidepressant. Unfortunately for them, trials suggested that clomipramine is in general no more effective than other antidepressants and has a worse side-effect profile, so the FDA turned down their application. In response, Geigy decided to test clomimpramine on the more specific disorder of obsessive compulsive disorder. In this case they were able to obtain satisfactory results and gained FDA approval to market the drug. This case demonstrates that whether a drug can be shown to be efficacious can depend on the population that is used for the trials.

The reverse case – where grouping disorders together is in the company's interest – can also occur. In *The Creation of Psychopharmacology*, Healy discusses the case of catatonia (2002: 272–5). Catatonia, Healy claims, is a distinct disorder from other types of schizophrenia, and furthermore it is a disorder for which there are cheap and effective treatments. However, as these treatments are old and unpatentable, the interests of pharmaceutical companies are best served by lumping catatonia with other types of schizophrenia. Thus clinical trials have looked at the action of antipsychotics on all types of schizophrenia rather than picking out patients who suffer from catatonia. Drugs companies sell more antipsychotics as a result, but patients suffering from catatonia are plausibly being denied effective treatments.

The choice of outcomes measures will also influence the apparent efficacy of the drug under test. The Hamilton Depression Rating Scale is one of the scales that is frequently used to rate the symptoms of depression. Healy notes that "Its items, which cover sleep and appetite, could not have been better designed to demonstrate the effects of tricyclic antidepressants like imipramine, which are somewhat sedative and appetite stimulant even in people who are not depressed" (1997: 98–9). On the other hand, one of the competitors to the Hamilton scale, the Beck Depression Inventory, focuses only on the cognitive aspects of depression. When such a scale is used to assess outcomes, cognitive therapy programmes thus appear particularly effective (*ibid.*: 99). Sponsors who want to show that a drug is effective can select outcomes criteria with an eye to increasing the likelihood of achieving positive results.

In an RCT the drug under test may either be compared with an existing treatment or with a placebo. Since the mid-1980s, the FDA has required that drugs are compared with placebo (*ibid.*: 133). In Europe it is more common for drugs to be compared with active treatments (Association of the British Pharmaceutical Industry (ABPI) 2003). Whether a drug is compared with placebo or with an active treatment, problems can arise. When a drug is tested against existing treatments this leaves open the possibility that neither drug may actually be better than placebo. In addition, it may be possible for the trial to be rigged in favour of the drug under test by prescribing the existing treatment in non-optimal doses (Angell 2005: 108). On the other hand, when drugs are tested against placebo the results may show that a drug is better than nothing (which satisfies the FDA), but they can provide no evidence that the drug is an improvement on existing medications (and, this after all is the question that prescribers and patients need addressed).

In addition, it is worth noting that RCTs can be very sensitive. With big enough sample sizes, RCTs can be used to unearth the slightest treatment effect. This makes it easier for drug companies to push drugs that are only marginally effective. A drug can be marketed as "being effective" for depression even when it does so little that its effects might pass unnoticed by an individual physician or patient. A recent review of the trials of SSRIs (drugs such as Prozac) that were used to gain FDA approval for these drugs found that the average difference between drug and placebo was only about two points of the sixty-two-point Hamilton Depression Rating Scale (Kirsch *et al.* 2002). This result is statistically significant, but still tiny. The authors conclude that "our data suggest that the effect of antidepressant drugs is very small and of questionable clinical significance". That the effects unearthed by RCTs can be very small means that it is harder for clinicians and users to confirm that the claimed benefits are genuine.

9.3.2 Publishing the right results

As we have seen, RCTs can be designed so that it is more likely that the results desired by the sponsors will be achieved. Often such measures will be sufficient to ensure that the company drug can be found to be "effective" for some particular condition. However, if the strategies outlined above fail to produce the desired results, pharmaceutical companies have other means of ensuring that only results favourable to them come to public attention.

When pharmaceutical companies apply for a licence to market a drug, they have to make available to the regulators all the data from the trials that they are using to demonstrate efficacy. In many cases the volume of data will be huge, and questions may be raised about the degree to which it is practically possible for it to be thoroughly reviewed. Nevertheless, at least the data summaries are scrutinized by the regulatory bodies that decide whether the drug can be marketed for particular indications. In both the US and in Europe, reviews of submitted trials are available to the public. These can be found online via the websites of the FDA and the European Medicine Evaluation Agency. Pharmaceutical companies have no control over the content of these official reports.

Manipulating the data that come to be published in medical journals is easier. In some cases pharmaceutical companies have prevented researchers from publishing the results of drug trials that are unfavourable to their product

(Bodenheimer 2000). Even if companies do not ban publication, there is in any case a tendency for researchers and journal editors to be less interested in "negative" results: papers that conclude only that a new drug is no better than an old one seem boring and so are less likely to be published (Gilbody & Song 2000). On the other hand, when a trial achieves positive results, sometimes multiple papers are published reporting this (*ibid.*). Such practices make it look as if many independent trials have found a drug to be efficacious when in actual fact all the results stem from one study.

Pharmaceutical companies can also increase the power that they have over trials by limiting the input of the academics that supposedly conduct them. The researchers that conduct trials are sometimes denied access to the full data sets that are produced (Healy 2003). This makes the researchers wholly reliant on the data that the company chooses to release to them.

In addition, a growing trend is for psychiatric research papers to be written by ghost-writers employed by pharmaceutical companies. The positive spin on this (see Lagnado 2003) is that it results in better-written papers being published more quickly. After all, many academics cannot write very well and others are too busy or disorganized to see projects through to completion. Ghost-writers can help such researchers. The ghost-writer edits and tidies work, and the "author" checks the final piece before publication. On such a picture, ghost-writers play a role in speeding research through to publication, but they do not actually shape the research.

On the other hand, the negative spin on ghost-writing is that it is part of a process via which pharmaceutical companies are gaining control of much psychiatric research. There is evidence that sometimes ghost-writers do not just assist researchers in the production of papers; sometimes ghost-writers do all the research. The "author" is then invited to add their name to a completed paper (see e.g. Healy 2004). Here, both pharmaceutical company and academic stand to benefit. The academic adds a publication to their record, which is important because academics are appointed and promoted on the basis of the works they have published. The pharmaceutical company benefits because a paper is published that praises their drug and appears to have been written by an independent and respected academic.

In the nature of things it is hard to form accurate estimates of the extent of ghost-writing. However there is some evidence that ghost-written papers can include those in the best journals with the best "authors". Furthermore, the results published in ghost-written papers consistently tend to be more favourable to pharmaceutical company products. David Healy and Dinah Cattell (2003) (also Healy 2004) have compared papers on Zoloft produced by one "medical information company" with papers produced independently. It is impossible to know the mix of agency versus academic input in the medical information company papers. All these papers will have involved ghost-writers, but in some the ghost-writers may have played a minor role. Still, the medical information company papers came out in the best journals, their "authors" were among the best-known researchers in the field and these papers received more citations. They also tended to report results that were more favourable for Zoloft.

Finally, it is worth noting that when a drug company designs a trial so that results favourable to its product are likely to be found, or manipulates the results that come to be reported, it is unlikely to get caught out. RCTs are necessarily big and expensive. This means that they are hard to replicate. As such a pharmaceutical company that succeeds in massaging the results of a trial is unlikely to get caught out by an independent replication.

On occasion it is suggested that the problems that we have seen with psychiatric research stem from the fact that pharmaceutical companies are commercial ventures. However, it is worth noting that the fact that pharmaceutical companies try to make money cannot be the sole cause of the problems. Much scientific research is conducted by commercial companies and in many areas this works well. Most of the technologies we use in daily living are developed by commercial ventures, and most of them are far better than their equivalents of twenty years ago (e.g. tennis rackets, waterproof clothing and cameras are all better than they were). The problem with psychiatric drugs is not merely that they are commercially produced, but that often the benefits of one drug over another are so subtle that they cannot be detected without the use of RCTs. As drug manufacturers control the RCTs, companies end up both developing new drugs and being the only ones who can tell whether the new drug actually is better. I suggest that it is this combination that causes problems.

9.4 Diagnosis of the problem

What has gone wrong with psychiatric research? Using ideas from Shapin and Schaffer's *Leviathan and the Air-Pump* (1985), in this section I shall suggest that the fundamental problem within psychiatric research is that methods for policing testimony have broken down. Simply put, the problem within psychiatric research is that investigators manipulate their research findings and they get away with it.

9.4.1 Shapin and Schaffer – the importance of policing testimony

Shapin and Schaffer's *Leviathan and the Air-Pump* is an important, well-known work in science studies. The book concerns a series of arguments between two seventeenth-century English natural philosophers: Thomas Hobbes and Robert Boyle. At one level Boyle and Hobbes argue about the existence of vacuums: Boyle believes they exist, Hobbes does not. At other levels Boyle and Hobbes also disagree about the importance of experimentation and, even more deeply, they disagree about the ways in which science should be politically organized.

In *Leviathan and the Air-Pump*, Shapin and Schaffer develop a number of claims, only one of which will concern us here. This is the claim that "Solutions to the problem of knowledge are solutions to the problem of social order" (1985: 332). The fundamental difficulty is that almost all knowledge depends on testimony. We can see and do little ourselves and so have to rely on the claims of others. However, only some others are trustworthy. Thus, before we can discover very much, the social problem of policing testimony must be solved. Shapin and Schaffer examine how Boyle developed techniques for disciplining witnesses and thus managed to shape the newly founded Royal Society into a body of experts that could produce credible claims.

Prior to Boyle, the older natural philosophy had been beset by difficulties because the problem of regulating witnesses had not been solved. Different individuals claimed to have seen different things, and there was no method for sorting reliable reports from unreliable reports. In Shapin and Schaffer's account, various innovations enabled Boyle's experimental programme to succeed in producing credible experimental claims. At the material level, skilful artisans, new techniques and large quantities of money made the construction of elaborate machines such as the air-pump possible. At the literary level, Boyle developed techniques for writing papers that enabled readers to reconstruct experiments in their "mind's eye". Finally, and of key interest to us here, Boyle succeeded in creating a new type of social organization within the Royal Society. For the first time the Royal Society made the laboratory a social space. Here a collection of expert observers together witnessed an experiment and then reached a consensus on what they had seen (*ibid*.: 57–8). Procedures were developed for recording the results of experiments. Following an experiment, the register of the Royal Society was "to be sign'd by a certain Number of the persons present, who have been present, and Witnesses of all the said proceedings, who, by Sub-scribing their Names, will prove undoubted Testimony" (*ibid*.: 58, quoting Hooke).

In theory, following publication of the report, witnesses to the experiment could be multiplied further. The experimental reports were written so as to facilitate replication. Thus, in principle, any researcher who wished could replicate the experiment for himself (*ibid*.: 59). It is worth noting, however, that even in Boyle's time replication was in actual fact rare. Boyle's equipment was exceedingly expensive, and getting it to work was very difficult.

Still, despite the problems with replication, Boyle to a large extent succeeded in policing the testimony that stemmed from the Royal Society. His method for policing testimony has the following features:

- named individuals witness the experiment;
- these individuals have something to lose if they are caught lying (their reputation for integrity);
- if the witnesses lie its possible (although in reality unlikely) that they might be caught because the experiment can be replicated; and
- the witnesses are multiplied.

Boyle's method is one way of regulating testimony but, as we shall see, there are also other means by which testimony can be policed.

9.4.2 Other solutions to the problem of policing testimony

Trusting to numbers and correction: Wikipedia

For a very different solution to the problem of policing testimony let us consider Wikipedia, the online encyclopedia. Launched in 2001, Wikipedia now contains over one million entries and receives as many as 14,000 hits per second (Schiff 2006). Authors are anonymous. Anyone can edit almost any of Wikipedia's entries (although a few pages, "Hitler" and "George Bush" among them, have special protection to prevent vandalism). Some of the resulting entries are very short, badly written and contain inaccuracies. However, over time, entries tend to be improved by other writers and evolve into comprehensive and fairly accurate sources of information. A recent study in *Nature* found that science articles in Wikipedia are of comparable accuracy to those found in the *Encyclopedia Britannica* (Wikipedia had four errors for every three in *Britannica*) (*ibid.*). The process by which Wikipedia entries evolve is explained in its replies to common objections:

> In all honesty, Wikipedia has a fair bit of well-meaning, but ill-informed and amateurish work. In fact, we welcome it – an amateurish article to be improved later is better than nothing. In any case, when new hands (particularly, experts on the subjects in question) arrive and go to work, the amateurish work is *usually* straightened out. Really egregious errors are fixed quickly by the thousands of people who read Wikipedia every day. (Wikipedia, n.d.)

Wikipedia is a free-for-all. The key to the accuracy of Wikipedia's entries is that mistakes can quickly be corrected by the vast numbers of people who read Wikipedia entries. A 2003 IBM study found that most cases of vandalism were fixed within five minutes (cited in Ebersbach *et al.* 2006: 27). Furthermore, cases of vandalism are reported to be lower than one might expect; one suggestion is that this is because vandalizing an entry is too easy to be any fun (*ibid.*).

Wikipedia is relatively new. Its success and accuracy have taken many commentators by surprise. It is probable that a Wikipedia can only work in certain social conditions. At the moment, Wikipedia articles get better over time. This must be because corrections are on average improvements: most of those who edit pages know what they are writing about and want to share their knowledge. Thus, sheer numbers of correctors is not enough. Under some conditions, edits would on average make the pages worse and the information would degenerate (consider, for example, what would happen if UK schoolchildren were regularly set the task of rewriting Wikipedia entries as part of a creative writing course). Still, Wikipedia shows that under certain social conditions, checking by anonymous but numerous others is sufficient to ensure the accuracy of testimony.

Trusting to micro-regulation and checking: food labels

For our final example, let us consider the claims made by the labels on food. Food labels make claims about fat content, salt content, place of origin and so on. As buyers we are rarely in a position to judge the accuracy of the claims that are made. If the fat content is actually 35 per cent instead of the reported 25 per cent we are rarely able to tell. What is more, those who sell food are strongly motivated to lie about the contents of their products. If they can get away with claiming that their burgers have a higher meat content and lower fat content than they really do they will be able to make more money. But, although consumers are not in a position to judge the accuracy of the claims that are made, and sellers are motivated to lie, for the most part the claims made on food labels are trustworthy. Here we will consider how micro-regulation and checking are employed to maintain the reliability of food labels.

The details about fat content, salt content and so on that are found on food labels derive from data produced in commercial laboratories. Some supermarkets have their own laboratories, and others contract out the testing that they require. For the supermarket to be able to give accurate information about the content of food it needs the laboratory reports on which it depends to be reliable. But here a problem emerges. The difficulty is that laboratory staff may be tempted to fabricate results. Particularly when one knows the results one can expect to get, it is easier to make up figures for salt content, meat content or whatever than to actually do the tests (I know this because I worked for a time in such a laboratory, and I was frequently tempted to make up results).

As anyone who has worked for a supermarket will know, supermarkets tend not to trust their employees. To stop their staff from stealing, supermarkets employ a range of mechanisms: uniforms may lack pockets; staff may have to leave bags in lockers; and so on. The supermarkets control behaviour that is easily observed (taking in bags) so that indirectly they can prevent behaviour that would otherwise be hard to observe (stealing). In the laboratories that test the food for large supermarkets micro-regulation is similarly employed. This time, however, the aim of micro-regulation is not to stop employees stealing, but rather to stop them lying.

Micro-regulation may be used to prevent the possibility of lying in numerous ways. For example, commercial laboratories may ban pencils and rough paper and insist that all calculations have to be written in ink in lab books with numbered pages. This makes it impossible to throw away the results of an analysis when they lead to the wrong answer.

Laboratories are micro-regulated to prevent staff from making up results. In addition, mechanisms are needed to stop the supermarkets from lying on food labels (once the laboratory staff have made accurate reports the supermarket may still be tempted to lie on the labels). At this stage, in the UK, deception by food-sellers is kept in check because the Foods Standards Agency runs independent tests on food to ensure that it contains what it says it contains. Sometimes these checks find that food has been falsely labelled. Recent investigations by the Foods Standards Agency have caught supermarkets selling minced meat and pizzas with higher fat content than that declared, for example, and have also found that much of the rice sold as "Basmati" rice is cheaper varieties (Food Standards Agency 2004a,b,c). Manufacturers who are caught cheating face bad publicity and risk prosecution. For example, the supermarket chain Tesco was in the news in 2005 because tests by the Food Standards Agency uncovered foods with higher than claimed salt levels (Fletcher & Ungoed-Thomas 2005). Thus, in the case of food labels, checking by an independent agency serves to keep deception at a minimum.

9.5 Returning to psychiatry

The examples of Boyle and the Royal Society, Wikipedia and food labelling, show us that policing testimony requires work. In general, informants cannot simply be trusted to give us the information that we need; rather, mechanisms have to be put in place to ensure that testimony is trustworthy. It is worth stressing that I do not think that researchers are particularly bad people: they are simply normal people. When placed in situations where they are motivated to mislead, and can get away with it, human beings have a tendency to be short with the truth. Suppose I ask my students whether they have done the seminar reading, or ask a fisherman how big a fish he caught last summer. I would be naive to fully trust the answers I receive.

Scientists are human rather than super-human, and also avoid telling the truth, or at least the whole truth, when it suits them. Whether scientists seek promotion, fame or money, reporting certain results will serve them better than others. When we ask scientists to tell us whether one drug is better than another, whether a cream really does remove wrinkles, or whether their research proposal is good value for money, we need there to be mechanisms in place for ensuring the reliability of their testimony before we can fully trust what they say. Depending on the methodologies that a science employs it may be more or less difficult to police testimony in that area. I suggest that certain features of RCT methodology have made the task of policing testimony in psychiatry particularly difficult.

Within psychiatry, various writers have recognized that there is currently a problem with the credibility of testimony and have proposed possible solutions. In looking at these we can see that they seek to use the various models that have worked elsewhere: some attempt to reinvigorate Boyle's model and make individual scientists trustworthy; others aim at increasing the extent to which published research findings can be checked by others; and others aim to impose additional micro-regulation that will force researchers to tell the truth.

9.5.1 Making the researchers trustworthy

Various proposals have sought to shore up traditional notions of scientific authorship; they have sought to make individual scientists responsible for ensuring the accuracy of reports. So, for example, the International Committee of Medical Journal Editors (ICMJE) states that each author should be able to "take public responsibility for appropriate portions of the content" and adds that "Some journals now also request that one or more authors, referred to as 'guarantors', be identified as the persons who take responsibility for the integrity of the work as a whole, from inception to published article" (ICMJE 2006).

The problem with expecting authors to be individually fully responsible for the contents of an entire paper is that it may not always be reasonable to expect an author to understand (let alone be in a position to judge) all aspects of a paper. In multidisciplinary research, researchers from different disciplines collaborate, so a psychiatrist may work with a statistician, or a social worker with an anthropologist. The whole point of such collaborations is that people from different disciplines can understand different material. If a psychiatrist could understand statistics, or the statistician could understand psychiatry, then they would not have needed to collaborate in the first place.

Having individual researchers take responsibility for portions of the paper will sometimes get around this problem. If, say, a clinician designed the trial and a statistician analysed the data, then it may be easy enough to attribute responsibility for each section of a paper. However, sometimes papers do not develop in a way that makes such attributions possible. If ten researchers work together and edit multiple drafts of a paper then each individual sentence may have been tweaked by ten people.

At this point we should pause and consider what the attribution of individual authorship is seeking to achieve. Mario Biagioli (1998) suggests that the felt need to attribute authorship, and thus responsibility to an individual, can be traced back to the days when authors who published heretical works could find themselves in trouble. As books could be heretical, and only named individuals could be punished for heresy, a named individual needed to take responsibility for every book. Biagioli suggests that the idea that an individual author is needed because someone must take responsibility for ensuring the accuracy of the contents of scientific papers echoes down to this day.

The thought that individual authorship is needed so that someone takes responsibility for a paper is widespread. However, there may be ways of ensuring that research is reliable without there being a named individual responsible for it. In some areas of science reliable research is produced by teams of workers, although the individual researchers remain anonymous. Consider weather forecasts, for example. Obviously some weather forecast services are better than others. However, the service as a whole, rather than an individual researcher, gains a reputation for reliability. There is no reason why qualities such as reliability, trustworthiness and so on should not be attributed to research groups as well as individuals. A group as a whole might develop a reputation for integrity, and be motivated to ensure that it managed to maintain this reputation. Under certain conditions, groups can be made responsible for ensuring that the work they produce is trustworthy. As such we can conclude that individual responsibility is not necessary to ensure the reliability of scientific research.

Another type of proposal that aims to make researchers trustworthy depends on removing the incentives for manipulating results. Marcia Angell has proposed setting up an independent Institute of Prescription Drug Trials (2005: 244–7). Angell suggests that drug companies could be required to fund this institute by a levy on their profits, but that they would have no say in the ways in which the trials were conducted. The institute would then commission independent researchers to run trials, and would make sure there was no incentive for them to produce one result rather than another.

It is worth noting that implementing Angell's suggestion would require a radical restructuring of psychiatric research. At present, independent researchers and institutions are hard to find. Prestigious universities universally maintain intimate links with industry (Schafer 2004). So too do scholarly and professional bodies: the APA gains a third of its income from pharmaceutical companies (Borenstein 2000). Representatives from the pharmaceutical companies even sit on the bodies that regulate the conduct of clinical trials (ICH 2000: 5). Currently, industry influence extends almost everywhere.

Still, if it were possible to institute, Angell's suggestion would doubtless remove some of the pressures on researchers. However, it is unlikely that it would solve the problems with testimony in psychiatric research on its own.

Healy notes that in some cases independent investigators have been found to engage in practices no less problematic than those employed by pharmaceutical companies (1997: 132). Researchers are not only motivated by money, but often also want to make a name for themselves, or are simply over-enthusiastic in pushing claims that they believe to be correct, and motives of these kinds can also lead to the distortion of published results. The problems that have emerged within psychiatric research are not caused simply by "evil drug companies"; rather, they emerge because systems of policing testimony have broken down. Investigators can be tempted to deceive for all kinds of reasons apart from commercial gain, and thus methods of ensuring the reliability of testimony are required irrespective of the researcher's affiliation.

9.5.2 Relying on micro-regulation and checking

Some writers have suggested that psychiatric research might be rendered reliable via various forms of micro-regulation. It is important to note that much regulation is already in place. Still, some commentators hold that current programmes of micro-regulation have failed, and so they suggest additional measures that they think might work.

The most common suggestion is that researchers should be forced to record the scope of all clinical trials at inception in a publicly available database. Indeed, the ICMJE has required that trials be logged on a database since 2004 (De Angelis *et al.* 2004). Journals that follow ICMJE guidelines (which include the *American Journal of Psychiatry* and the *British Journal of Psychiatry*) now refuse to publish papers stemming from non-logged trials. It is possible to view the database of trials maintained by the US National Institute of Health at http://clinicaltrials.gov. The principle role of such databases is to provide a public record of all trials. Hopefully, this will make it harder for companies to hide trial results when the findings go against commercial interests. It will also make it difficult for the same trial to be reported in multiple papers (thus giving the misleading impression that a number of different studies have found the same result).

Investigators are also supposed to use the database to log details of the primary and secondary outcomes that will be used to judge whether the drug under test is efficacious. This should help prevent the practice of "data dredging", where investigators with a generally disappointing drug look at multiple outcome measures in the hope of finding at least some that indicate advantages. At present the degree to which logged trials comply with the spirit of specifying prospective outcome measures varies. If one looks at trials that are investigating interventions for depression, for example, some give much more detail regarding outcome measures than others. Thus trial NCT00143091 states that its primary outcome will be the "Change from baseline in HAM-D (17) [the Hamilton Depression Rating

Scale] at the week 6 visit". In contrast, and less helpfully, trial NCT00146523 will use as a primary outcome "The change in a measure of psychosis". A recent editorial in the *New England Journal of Medicine* notes that the quality of information recorded in the database has improved in recent years, and is hopeful that this trend will continue (Drazen & Zarin 2007).

It is worth noting that using replication to ensure the trustworthiness of reported results has only limited potential. Unfortunately it is in the nature of RCTs to be big, complex and expensive. However, although it is hard to replicate entire trials, checking can be employed to ensure that at least some stages of the trial have been performed correctly. The FDA currently has inspectors who go to some clinical trial sites and inspect study documents and clinical notes to check that the study is being conducted as it should (Healy 1997: 133; Katz 2004). However, as an employee of the FDA accepts, "resource limitations preclude detailed inspections of most of the clinical data generated" (Katz 2004: 310). At present pharmaceutical companies tend to be unwilling to release the raw data from drug trials. But, if they were made to do so, then independent investigators could at least check that the data had been analysed correctly (Healy & Cattell 2003).

9.6 Conclusion

Various practices have recently been introduced that will hopefully improve the reliability of drug trial papers. The extent to which they will prove successful remains to be seen.

The example of industry-run RCTs illustrates how a new type of social epistemology is needed and how it might differ from traditional epistemology. Traditional epistemology has assumed that agents are competent and honest. Reflecting this tradition, most of the philosophical literature on RCTs assumes that researchers can be trusted not to manipulate the studies they perform. Given such an assumption, RCT techniques seem to be a good idea. However, if we abandon this assumption and take on board evidence that shows that researchers are not maximally honest, then RCTs appear in a different light.

Various features of RCTs make them vulnerable to manipulation: most obviously they are hard to replicate because they are so expensive and so sensitive. In addition, difficult decisions have to be made, for example, regarding the subject population and measures of effectiveness, and these decisions can be made with the intention of maximizing the chances of getting positive results for the drug under test. Thus, when one takes on board the possibility that researchers may have reason to massage their results, RCTs no longer appear the obvious choice for assessing new therapies.

I conclude that if epistemologists remember that scientists are real people rather than ideal truth-seekers then this will make a difference to the kinds of methods they will recommend. For example, in a large RCT, replicability is sacrificed in the pursuit of increased sensitivity: larger trials are more sensitive but also harder to replicate, because they are expensive. If one is advising ideal knowledge-seekers then such a trade-off may be justified. After all, if the best possible trial is run by the best possible people, replication will be unnecessary. However, as soon as one begins to doubt the trustworthiness of researchers, the extent to which an experiment can be replicated becomes an issue of key importance. A social epistemology would pay more attention to the extent to which different methods can be manipulated by those who are not primarily interested in knowledge-seeking, and would consider how science might best be socially organized so that socially situated actors can be encouraged to discover and share truths. The example of RCTs in psychiatry shows that such a social epistemology is badly needed.

10. Conclusion

We have focused on four features of psychiatry that distinguish it from many other sciences: (i) the subject matter of psychiatry is contested; (ii) psychiatry employs particular modes of explanation; (iii) mental health professionals work within multiple different theoretical frameworks; and (iv) psychiatry is problematically shaped by values and interests.

In Chapters 2 and 3 I examined the nature of mental illness. I concluded that the antipsychiatrists are mistaken, and that mental illness is no myth. When it comes to providing a positive account of mental disorder, the jury is still out. At present there are multiple accounts of disorder being developed, and it is unclear which, if any, will prove successful. Still, a consensus is emerging on some fronts. Most agree that mental and physical disorders cannot be cleanly distinguished. In addition, it looks likely that determining whether a condition is a disorder involves value judgements. Still, even if value judgements are involved in determining whether a condition is a disorder, projects that seek to investigate the causes and natural history of particular conditions can be properly scientific.

With the subject matter of psychiatry ensured, in Chapters 4 and 5 we examined two types of explanation that are particularly common in psychiatry. Chapter 4 focused on "natural-history style" explanations. These explanations work by identifying the natural kind to which an individual belongs. I argued that at least some types of mental disorder are plausibly natural kinds, and that the use of such explanations in psychiatry is thus justified. To the extent that psychiatry makes use of natural-history style explanations it can be considered alongside other natural historical sciences, such as geology and botany. Chapter 5 focused on the use of individual case histories. I used simulation-based accounts of folk-psychological understanding to develop an account of how such case histories work. I argued that case histories work by providing us with the scaffolding necessary to simulate the thoughts of another, and discussed possible limits to this process. To the extent that such case histories can be regarded as a species of simulation-based explanation, psychiatry can be considered alongside all sciences that use simulations to explain.

Characteristically, within psychiatry there is agreement over little, and multiple schools and theories compete. Chapters 6 and 7 considered relationships between the different theoretical frameworks within psychiatry. In Chapter 6 I argued that psychiatry is a multi-paradigm science. Kuhn claimed that communication between paradigms is problematic, but I suggested that in practice communication problems can be overcome via the construction of contact languages and through shared direct contact with patients. Chapter 7 looked at reductionism within psychiatry. At the metaphysical level, the big questions concern the mind–brain relationship. Multiple accounts of the mind are on the philosophical marketplace, and I did not attempt to solve the vexed question of the relationship between mind and body. I argued that as long as one stays clear of eliminative materialism, talk of the mind is safe, and that psychiatric research can continue whichever philosophical account of the mind turns out to be correct. At the epistemic level, I examined arguments developed by Fodor and Davidson that attempt to show that psychological theories cannot be reduced to theories at a lower level. I argued that the implications of their arguments for psychiatry are limited, and that reductionist projects within psychiatry may prove successful.

Chapters 8 and 9 looked at the ways in which psychiatry is problematically shaped by values and interests. Chapter 8 examined the ways in which psychiatry is a value-laden science. I argued that psychiatry is affected by values at every stage of enquiry. Plausibly, other sciences are also value-laden in similar ways. Still, as long as a research area involves diverse researchers, and facilitates free criticism, many of the problems caused by value-ladenness can be overcome. Researchers with different viewpoints will be able to spot problems that others have overlooked, and once a researcher has spotted a problem others can come to appreciate their arguments regardless of their initial outlook. Chapter 9 looked at the use of RCTs to evaluate psychiatric treatments. I argued that various features of RCTs make them vulnerable to manipulation by parties with an interest in ensuring that a trial produces a particular outcome. The example of industry-run RCTs illustrates how a new type of social epistemology is needed and how it might differ from traditional epistemology. Such a social epistemology would pay more attention to the extent to which different methods can be manipulated by those who are not primarily interested in knowledge-seeking, and would consider how science might best be socially organized so that socially situated actors can be encouraged to discover and share truths

By focusing on the four themes of the book, I have shown that psychiatry is similar enough to other sciences for ideas from the philosophy of science to be helpful in solving conceptual problems within psychiatry. Also, I have demonstrated that psychiatry is simultaneously different enough from other sciences for an investigation of psychiatry to enable old problems in the philosophy of science to be viewed from a new and fruitful angle.

Notes

1. Introduction: psychiatry and philosophy of science

1. Those interested in the policies of hospital closure might consult P. Barham, *Closing the Asylum* (Harmondsworth: Penguin, 1992).
2. For a history see P. Campbell, "The History of the User Movement in the United Kingdom", in *Mental Health Matters: A Reader*, T. Heller, J. Reynolds, R. Gomm *et al.* (eds), 218–25 (Basingstoke: Macmillan, 1996).
3. For a flavour of the debates see P. Calloway, C. Denman, N. Hymas and C. Lawton, "Patients and Clients", *British Journal of Psychiatry* **178** (2001), 276.
4. For a recent discussion within psychiatry of Popper and the scientific status of psychoanalysis see D. Grant and E. Harari, "Psychoanalysis, Science and the Seductive Theory of Karl Popper", *Australian and New Zealand Journal of Psychiatry* **39** (2005), 446–52.

2. The nature of mental illness 1: is mental illness a myth?

1. See T. Gendler and J. Hawthorne, The Real Guide to Fake Barns: A Catalogue of Gifts for your Epistemic Enemies", *Philosophical Studies* **124** (2005), 331–52, for an up-to-date discussion of the problems caused by Fake Barns and similar knowledge defeaters.
2. See various papers and responses in *History of the Human Sciences* **3**(1) and **3**(3) (1990) for discussion of the historical accuracy of Foucault's claims and of the differences between the two versions of his work.

3. The nature of mental illness 2: if mental disorders exist, what are they?

1. For details of the 1970s debates over homosexuality see R. Bayer, *Homosexuality and American Psychiatry* (New York: Basic Books, 1981).
2. A short and clear summary of the account is provided in K. W. M. Fulford, T. Thornton and G. Graham, *Oxford Textbook of Philosophy and Psychiatry* (Oxford: Oxford University Press, 2006), 128–33.

4. Explanations in psychiatry 1: natural-history based explanations

1. See D. Murphy, *Psychiatry in the Scientific Image* (Cambridge, MA: MIT Press, 2006) for a discussion of the use of some other types of explanation in psychiatry, in particular those that make use of non-strict causal laws, the box-style models of cognitive sciences and also evolutionary explanations.
2. Murphy, *Psychiatry in the Scientific Image*, and L. Reznek, *The Philosophical Defence of Psychiatry* (London: Routledge, 1991) have similar views of explanations that are based on classification. Murphy notes that "classification can reflect causal discrimination in the absence of causal understanding" (*Psychiatry in the Scientific Image*, 319) (i.e. we can know that two kinds are causally different, even if we do not know exactly how they are different), and Reznek thinks that classification can provide at least the promise of an explanation (*The Philosophical Defence of Psychiatry*, 187–9) (although he holds that while the underlying nature of a kind remains unspecified we do not have an explanation of the behaviour of members of the kind but only a promise of an explanation).
3. These studies are summarized in T. Widiger, A. Frances, H. Pincus *et al.* (eds), *DSM-IV Sourcebook, vol. 1* (Washington, DC: American Psychiatric Association, 1994), *vol. 2* (1996), *vol. 3* (1997).
4. The links between kinds, laws, inductive inferences and explanation are clearly explored in A. Bird, *Philosophy of Science* (London: UCL Press, 1998), ch. 3, and also in R. Boyd, "Realism, Anti-foundationalism and the Enthusiasm for Natural Kinds", *Philosophical Studies* **61** (1991), 127–48 and T. Wilkerson, *Natural Kinds* (Aldershot: Avebury, 1995).
5. McGinn himself is not a functionalist, but he presents these arguments from a functionalist's perspective. G. Botterill and P. Carruthers, *The Philosophy of Psychology* (Cambridge: Cambridge University Press, 1999), 39, also suggest that the multiple realizability of psychological kinds means that they cannot be natural kinds.
6. The first five papers in *Schizophrenia Research* **17** (1995) are devoted to the question of whether schizophrenia is a heterogeneous disorder: see L. E. DeLisi and H. A. Nasrallah, "Current Controversies in Schizophrenia Reaearch. I: Is Schizophrenia a Heterogeneous Disorder?", 133; T. J. Crow, "A Continuum of Psychosis, One Human Gene, and Not Much Else – the Case for Homogeneity", 135–45; T. E. Goldberg and D. R. Weinberger, "A Case Against Subtyping in Schizophrenia", 147–52; A. G. Cardno and A. E. Farmer, "The Case For or Against Heterogeneity in the Etiology of Schizophrenia: the Genetic Evidence", 153–9; and M. T. Tsuang and S. V. Faraone, "The Case for Heterogeneity in the Etiology of Schizophrenia", 161–75.
7. For more on links between classification in psychiatry and drug marketing see D. Healy, *The Antidepressant Era* (Cambridge, MA: Harvard University Press, 1997).

5. Explanations in psychiatry 2: individual case histories

1. For a selection of classic articles see P. Carruthers and P. Smith, *Theories of Theories of Mind* (Cambridge: Cambridge University Press, 1996). For a recent summary of the current state of play see A. Goldman, *Simulating Minds* (Oxford: Oxford University Press, 2006).
2. This claim is also made by R. Sorensen, "Self-strengthening Empathy", *Philosophy and Phenomenological Research* **58** (1998), 75–98.
3. For more on how our ability to empathize might be limited by the aversive affect produced see M. Hoffman, *Empathy and Moral Development: Implications for Caring and Justice* (Cambridge: Cambridge University Press, 2000).
4. This comes out particularly clearly in J. Heal, *Mind, Reason and Imagination* (Cambridge: Cambridge University Press, 2003) and R. Gordan, "Folk Psychology as

Simulation", in *Folk Psychology*, M. Davies & T. Stone (eds), 60–73 (Oxford: Blackwell, 1995).

5. K. Stueber, "The Psychological Basis of Historical Explanation", *History and Theory* **41** (2002), 25–42, focuses on historical explanation and also suggests that we can think of *Verstehen* as working via simulation.
6. In Karl Jaspers, "Causal and 'Meaningful' Connections Between Life History and Psychosis", J. Hoenig (trans.), in *Themes and Variations in European Psychiatry*, S. Hirsch & M. Shepherd (eds), 80–93 (Bristol: Wright, [1913] 1974), Jaspers writes that "Meaningful connexions are ideally typical connexions" – in a sense allied to Weber's ideal types – but it is obscure exactly what Jaspers is suggesting here.
7. This point is also made by I. Ravenscroft, "What is it Like to be Someone Else? Simulation and Empathy", *Ratio* **11** (1998), 170–85, and Hoffman, *Empathy and Moral Development*.

6. Relations between theories 1: when paradigms meet

1. In *The Structure of Scientific Revolutions* (Chicago, IL: University of Chicago Press, 1970), 178 and 209, Kuhn allows that occasionally a developed science may possess competing schools, and he suggests that immature sciences may have multiple paradigms (*ibid.*: 179). For our project here, considering whether and how inter-paradigm communication is possible, whether or not Kuhn holds that sometimes there are multiple paradigms within a sub-discipline does not matter.
2. J. Molyneaux, "Interprofessional Teamworking: What Makes Teams Work Well?", *Journal of Interprofessional Care* **15** (2001), 29–35, also notes that multidisciplinary teams work best when members are of equal status. N. Stanley, B. Penhale, D. Riordan *et al.*, "Working on the Interface: Identifying Professional Responses to Families with Mental Health and Child-care Needs", *Health and Social Care in the Community* **11** (2003), 208–18, esp. 213, note how the comparatively high status of medics results in communication problems with other professionals.
3. In his study of mental health professionals in Argentina, A. Lakoff, *Pharmaceutical Reason: Knowledge and Value in Global Psychiatry* (Cambridge: Cambridge University Press, 2005) similarly found that biologically oriented psychiatrists and psychoanalysts consider each other to pose a risk to patients. In an interesting twist, local conditions meant that here biologically oriented psychiatrists could accuse analysts of over-medicating patients. In Argentina, Lacanian psychoanalysts work in public mental hospitals. They tend to diagnose psychosis where a biologically oriented psychiatrist might diagnose bipolar disorder, and as a consequence they prescribe antipsychotics where a biologically oriented psychiatrist might prescribe mood-stabilizers. One of Lakoff's respondents thought "there was a public health disaster in Argentina, in which large numbers of patients were kept sedated and unnecessarily institutionalized through misdiagnosis and the wrong medication … this was the scandal of treating hospitalized patients psychoanalytically" (*ibid.*: 98). Lakoff's analytic respondents also had a dim view of biologically oriented psychiatrists, and considered their treatments to be superficial.
4. In his study of mental health services in Argentina, Lakoff (2005) similarly reports that analysts and biologically oriented psychiatrists cultivate different styles. He found that "the urbane, professorial habitus of the analysts contrasted with the harried disrepair of the self-consciously biomedical psychiatrists" (*Pharmaceutical Reason*, 82).
5. Family therapists constitute the main group who have problems with the assumptions that are implicit in the DSM. Many family therapists do not consider mental disorders to be the result of individual problems. Instead they think that mental disorders

are symptomatic of structural familial problems. So they have problems with the DSM because it provides diagnoses for individuals rather than groups.

6. Those who are familiar with Quine's work can note that the problems associated with translating between Quine's conceptual schemes are importantly different from the problems associated with translating between Kuhnian paradigms. Quine thinks that there are multiple translations between conceptual schemes, while Kuhn thinks there is no way to translate between paradigms.
7. Causal accounts of reference are most closely linked with S. Kripke, *Naming and Necessity*, rev. edn (Oxford: Blackwell, 1980) and H. Putnam, "Is Semantics Possible?", in *Mind, Language and Reality*, 139–52 (Cambridge: Cambridge University Press, 1970).
8. The difference this makes can be seen in A. Stanton and M. Schwartz, *The Mental Hospital* (New York: Basic Books, 1954), 86, where a table of improvement rates compares assessments by analysts (who value insight) and by administrative psychiatrists (who value getting patients home and working).
9. In the VA's case "compliance was mandated by software that would not permit a record to be signed out without a GAF score". Unfortunately for the VA, the original GAF system allowed for a "0" to be recorded in cases when there was insufficient information for a rating to be made. Soon the VA found that practitioners were giving a "0" in most cases. Faced with this "non-compliance in spirit" the VA removed the "0" score (Veterans Health Administration, *Instituting Global Assessment of Function (GAF) Scores in Axis V for Mental Health Patients*, VHA Directive 97-059, 25 November 1997, www.avapl.org/gaf/gaf.html).

7. Relations between theories 2: reductionisms

1. J. Kim, *Supervenience and Mind* (Cambridge: Cambridge University Press, 1993), 309–35, also argues that multiple realization may be compatible with species-level reductions.
2. For a detailed discussion of how such reductions might be worked out in practice see Murphy, *Psychiatry in the Scientific Image*.

8. Managing values and interests 1: psychiatry as a value-laden science

1. For studies of gender and psychiatry see E. Lunbeck, *The Psychiatric Persuasion* (Princeton, NJ: Princeton University Press, 1994), on race see S. Fernando, *Mental Health, Race and Culture*, 2nd edn (Basingstoke: Palgrave Macmillan, 2002).
2. Further examples of the ways in which values shape the interpretation of results can be found in S. Gould, *The Mismeasure of Man* (Harmondsworth: Penguin, 1981), 217–21. Gould discusses how Lewis Madison Terman managed to interpret statistics from IQ tests conducted on army recruits in line with his prior assumptions. R. Richardson, "Biology and Ideology: The Interpenetration of Science and Values", *Philosophy of Science* **51** (1984), 396–420, also notes that explanations that fit in with our expectations are subjected to less scrutiny.
3. For discussion see A. Chappell, "Emergence of Participatory Methodology in Learning Difficulty Research: Understanding the Context", *British Journal of Learning Disabilities* **28** (2000), 38–43, and J. Walmsley, "Normalisation, Emancipatory Research and Inclusive Research in Learning Disability", *Disability and Society* **16** (2001), 187–205. For an example of a research paper by a person with learning disabilities see S. Aspis, "Self-advocacy for People with Learning Difficulties: Does it Have a Future?", *Disability and Society* **12** (1997), 647–54.

4. See, for example, A. Thomas and S. Sillen, *Racism and Psychiatry* (New York: Brunner/Mazel, 1972), which discusses some of the papers examined in this chapter.

9. Managing values and interests 2: big business and judging treatments

1. For discussion of the ethical problems that surround RCTs see *Journal of Medical Ethics* **30**(2) (2004), a special issue devoted to these topics.
2. In his study of mental health in Argentina, Lakoff, *Pharmaceutical Reason*, esp. 8–9, 84, also found that analysts see drugs as acting on symptoms.
3. Lakoff also found that distinct professional groups disagreed about what counted as a successful treatment. Here the disagreement was between traditional analysts and those who provided brief therapy. Disputes arose: "did efficacy simply mean improvement on standardized measures of functionality? Or did therapy strive for something deeper and more profound?" (*Pharmaceutical Reason*, 124).
4. See, for example, C. Knowles, *Bedlam on the Streets* (London: Routledge, 2000) on drug use in Canadian foster homes for the mentally ill.
5. For reviews see D. Chambless and T. Ollendick, "Empirically Supported Psychological Interventions: Controversies and Evidence", *Annual Review of Psychology* **52** (2001), 685–716, and A. Roth and P. Fonagy, *What Works for Whom?* (New York: Guilford, 1996).

Further reading

Full bibliographic details are given in the bibliography.

Those who would like to read more about the philosophy of science could usefully start with Alan Chalmers's *What is This Thing Called Science?* (1999). This book is well written and accessible, and is widely used in teaching introductory philosophy of science courses.

Recommending texts in the philosophy of psychiatry is more difficult, as until very recently the area has been neglected. Currently, two comprehensive sources are available. *The Philosophy of Psychiatry* (2004), edited by Jennifer Radden, is a big reference book that contains articles on all areas of the philosophy of psychiatry. Alternatively, readers could try Bill Fulford, Tim Thornton and George Graham's *Oxford Textbook of Philosophy and Psychiatry* (2006). This is a huge textbook that thoroughly introduces all the main issues in the philosophy of psychiatry. It comes with a useful CD of accompanying readings.

On the nature of mental illness

Works by the antipsychiatrists are widely available and fairly easy to read. Thomas Szasz's best-known work is *The Myth of Mental Illness* (1961). R. D. Laing's work is highly variable. His most accessible work (with A. Esterson) is *Sanity, Madness and the Family* (1970). Foucault is quite hard, but worth the effort. *History of Madness* (2006) is very long, so most readers should choose to stick with *Madness and Civilisation* (1971).

All of the above works are fairly old. For more recent critiques of psychiatry, readers might try Pat Bracken and Phil Thomas's *Postpsychiatry* (2005). Alternatively, the Critical Psychiatry Network has many papers and links to other works on their website: www.critpsynet.freeuk.com.

Of works that seek to defend psychiatry from antipsychiatric complaints the most accessible is Laurie Reznek's *The Philosophical Defence of Psychiatry* (1991).

Readers who are interested in the nature of disorder might start with Laurie Reznek's *The Nature of Disease* (1987), which is short and well written. Useful collections of articles can be found in *Concepts of Health and Disease* (1981) and *Health, Disease, and Illness* (2004), both edited by Arthur Caplan *et al.*, and *What is Disease?* (1997), edited by James Humber and Robert Almeder.

On explanation in psychiatry

Works on explanation in psychiatry tend to be challenging. Dominic Murphy's *Psychiatry in the Scientific Image* (2006) looks at classification and forms of explanation in psychiatry. My *Classifying Madness* (2005) and John Sadler's *Values and Psychiatric Diagnosis* (2005) examine philosophical issues surrounding classification in psychiatry.

On relations between theories

Readers interested in paradigms should start with Thomas Kuhn's *The Structure of Scientific Revolutions* (1970). Tanya Luhrmann's *Of Two Minds* (2000) is among the most interesting books looking at differences between different groups of mental health professionals. The key text on contact languages is Peter Galison's *Image and Logic* (1997). This is an extremely long book, but Chapter 9 is the most relevant.

Readers wanting an introduction to different accounts of the relation between the mind and the brain should start with any of the many introductory textbooks in the philosophy of mind. Possibilities include Robert Kirk's *Mind and Body* (2003). Derek Bolton and Jonathan Hill's *Mind, Meaning and Mental Disorder* (1996) examines causal and meaningful explanations of behaviour in psychiatry. It is quite difficult but may be of interest. Dominic Murphy's *Psychiatry in the Scientific Image* (2006) looks at models of reduction that might be appropriate for psychiatry.

Managing values and interests

Some of the best material on value-ladenness in science can be found in works on the feminist philosophy of science. Helen Longino's *Science as Social Knowledge* (1990) is especially recommended. For readers looking for other examples of value-ladenness in science, Stephen Jay Gould's *The Mismeasure of Man* (1981) is an accessible book that examines the ways in which debates over intelligence quotient have been shaped by the values of the participants.

Those interested in the links between pharmaceutical companies and psychiatry should consult work by David Healy: *The Antidepressant Era* (1997) or *The Creation of Psychopharmacology* (2002). Alternatively, Marcia Angell's *The Truth About the Drug Companies* (2005) is more general and easier to read.

Bibliography

Association of the British Pharmaceutical Industry (ABPI) 2003. *Clinical Trials – Developing New Medicines*, www.abpi.org.uk/publications/briefings/clinical_brief.pdf

Akeret, R. 1995. *The Man Who Loved A Polar Bear*. Harmondsworth: Penguin.

Akiskal, H. 1998. "Toward a Definition of Generalised Anxiety Disorder as an Anxious Temperament Type". *Acta Psychiatrica Scandinavica Supplement* **393**: 66–73.

American Journal of Insanity 1844. "Number of the Insane and Idiotic, with brief notices of the Lunatic Asylums of the United States". *American Journal of Insanity* **1**: 78–88.

American Journal of Insanity 1851. "Startling Facts from the Census (reprinted article from the New York Observer)". *American Journal of Insanity* **8**: 153–5.

American Psychiatric Association (APA) 1952. *Diagnostic and Statistical Manual: Mental Disorders*. Washington, DC: American Psychiatric Association.

American Psychiatric Association (APA) 1980. *Diagnostic and Statistical Manual of Mental Disorders*, 3rd edn. Washington, DC: American Psychiatric Association.

American Psychiatric Association (APA) 1994. *Diagnostic and Statistical Manual of Mental Disorders*, 4th edn. Washington, DC: American Psychiatric Association.

Angell, M. 2005. *The Truth About the Drug Companies*. New York: Random House.

Ashcroft, R. 2004. "Current Epistemological Problems in Evidence Based Medicine". *Journal of Medical Ethics* **30**: 131–5.

Aspis, S. 1997. "Self-advocacy for People with Learning Difficulties: Does it Have a Future?". *Disability and Society* **12**: 647–54.

Baker, C., M. Johnsrud, M. Crismon, R. Rosenheck & S. Woods 2003. "Quantitative Analysis of Sponsorship Bias in Economic Studies of Antidepressants". *The British Journal of Psychiatry* **183**: 498–506.

Banyard, P. 1999. *Controversies in Psychology*. London: Routledge.

Barham, P. 1992. *Closing the Asylum*. Harmondsworth: Penguin.

Barnes, M. & P. Shardlow 1996. "Identity Crisis: Mental Health User Groups and the 'Problem' of Identity". In *Exploring the Divide*, C. Barnes & G. Mercer (eds), 114–34. Leeds: Disability Press.

Bayer, R. 1981. *Homosexuality and American Psychiatry*. New York: Basic Books.

Bevis, W. 1921. "Psychological Traits of the Southern Negro with Observations as to some of his Psychoses". *American Journal of Psychiatry* **78**: 69–78.

Biagioli, M. 1998. "The Instability of Authorship: Credit and Responsibility in Contemporary Biomedicine". *FASEB Journal* **12**(1): 3–16.

Bird, A. 1998. *Philosophy of Science*. London: UCL Press.

Blasi, V., A. Young, A. Tansy, S. Petersen, A. Snyder & M. Corbetta 2002. "Word Retrieval Learning Modulates Right Frontal Cortex in Patients with Left Frontal Damage". *Neuron* **36**: 159–70.

Block, N. 1978. "Troubles with Functionalism". *Minnesota Studies in the Philosophy of Science*, vol. IX, C. Savage (ed.), 261–325. Minneapolis, MN: University of Minnesota Press.

Bodenheimer, T. 2000. "Uneasy Alliance – Clinical Investigators and the Pharmaceutical Industry". *New England Journal of Medicine* **342**: 1539–44.

Bogen, J. 1988. "Comments on 'The Sociology of Knowledge about Child Abuse'". *Noûs* **22**: 65–6.

Bolton, D. & J. Hill 1996. *Mind, Meaning and Mental Disorder*. Oxford: Oxford University Press.

Boorse, C. 1975. "On the Distinction Between Disease and Illness". *Philosophy and Public Affairs* **5**: 49–68.

Boorse, C. 1976. "What a Theory of Mental Health Should Be". *Journal of Social Behaviour* **6**: 61–84.

Boorse, C. 1977. "Health as a Theoretical Concept". *Philosophy of Science* **44**: 542–73.

Boorse, C. 1997. "A Rebuttal on Health". In *What is Disease?*, J. Hunter & R. Almeder (eds), 1–134. Totowa, NJ: Humana Press.

Borenstein, D. 2000. "Pharmaceutical Companies". *Psychiatric News* **35** (17 November): 9.

Botterill, G. & P. Carruthers 1999. *The Philosophy of Psychology*. Cambridge: Cambridge University Press.

Boyd, R. 1991. "Realism, Anti-foundationalism and the Enthusiasm for Natural Kinds". *Philosophical Studies* **61**: 127–48.

Bracken, P. & P. O'Sullivan 2001. "The Invisibility of Irish Migrants in British Health Research". *Irish Studies Review* **9**: 41–51.

Bracken, P. & P. Thomas 2005. *Postpsychiatry: Mental Health in a Postmodern World*. Oxford: Oxford University Press.

Bräunig, P., G. Shugar & S. Krüger 1996. "An Investigation of the Self-report Manic Inventory as a Diagnostic and Severity Scale for Mania". *Comprehensive Psychiatry* **37**: 52–5.

Breggin, P. 1993. *Toxic Psychiatry*. London: HarperCollins. First published 1991.

Browne, J. 1996. "Biogeography and Empire". In *Cultures of Natural History*, N. Jardine, J. Secord & E. Spary (eds), 305–21. Cambridge: Cambridge University Press.

Burchnall, K. 2006. "Are there Kuhnian Paradigms in Psychology?". Unpublished MA essay, Lancaster University.

Cabaniss, D. 2001. "Beyond Dualism: Psychoanalysis and Medication in the 21st Century". *Bulletin of the Menninger Clinic* **65**: 160–70.

Calloway, P., C. Denman, N. Hymas & C. Lawton 2001. "Patients and Clients". *British Journal of Psychiatry* **178**: 276.

Campbell, P. 1996. "The History of the User Movement in the United Kingdom". In *Mental Health Matters: A Reader*, T. Heller, J. Reynolds, R. Gomm *et al.* (eds), 218–25. Basingstoke: Macmillan.

Campbell, J. 2001. "Rationality, Meaning and the Analysis of Delusion". *Philosophy, Psychiatry, & Psychology* **8**: 89–100.

Caplan, A. L., H. T. Engelhardt Jr., & J. J. McCartney (eds) 1981. *Concepts of Health and Disease: Interdisciplinary Perspectives*. Reading, MA: Addison-Wesley.

Caplan, A. L., J. J. McCartney & D. A. Sisti (eds) 2004. *Health, Disease, and Illness: Concepts in Medicine*. Washington, DC: Georgetown University Press.

Cardno, A. G. & A. E. Farmer 1995. "The Case For or Against Heterogeneity in the Etiology of Schizophrenia: the Genetic Evidence". *Schizophrenia Research* **17**: 153–9.

Carruthers, P. & P. Smith 1996. *Theories of Theories of Mind*. Cambridge: Cambridge University Press.

Chalmers, A. 1999. *What is This Thing Called Science?*, 3rd edn. Milton Keynes: Open University Press.

Chalmers, D. 1996. *The Conscious Mind*. Oxford: Oxford University Press.

Chambless, D. & T. Ollendick 2001. "Empirically Supported Psychological Interventions: Controversies and Evidence". *Annual Review of Psychology* **52**: 685–716.

Chappell, A. 2000. "Emergence of Participatory Methodology in Learning Difficulty Research: Understanding the Context". *British Journal of Learning Disabilities* **28**: 38–43.

Churchland, P. 1981. "Eliminative Materialism and the Propositional Attitudes". *Journal of Philosophy* **78**: 67–90.

Collins, H. & T. Pinch 1993. *The Golem – What Everyone Should Know About Science*. Cambridge: Cambridge University Press.

Colombo, A., G. Bendelow, B. Fulford & S. Williams 2003. "Evaluating the Influence of Implicit Models of Mental Disorder on Processes of Shared Decision Making within Community-based Multi-disciplinary Teams". *Social Science and Medicine* **56**: 1557–70.

Cooper, R. 2002. "Disease". *Studies in History and Philosophy of Biological and Biomedical Sciences* **33**: 263–82.

Cooper, R. 2004. "Why Hacking is Wrong about Human Kinds". *British Journal for the Philosophy of Science* **55**: 73–85.

Cooper, R. 2005. *Classifying Madness: A Philosophical Examination of the Diagnostic and Statistical Manual of Mental Disorders*. Dordrecht: Springer.

Crow, T. J. 1995. "A Continuum of Psychosis, One Human Gene, and Not Much Else – the Case for Homogeneity". *Schizophrenia Research* **17**: 135–45.

Cummins, R. 1975. "Functional Analysis". *Journal of Philosophy* **72**: 741–65.

Davidson, D. 1973/4. "On the Very Idea of a Conceptual Scheme". *Proceedings of the American Philosophical Association* **47**: 5–20.

Davidson, D. 1980a. "Mental Events". In his *Essays on Actions and Events*, 207–27. Oxford: Oxford University Press. First published 1970.

Davidson, D. 1980b. "Psychology as Philosophy". In his *Essays on Actions and Events*, 229–39. Oxford: Oxford University Press. First published 1974.

Davidson, D. 1982. "Paradoxes of Irrationality". In *Philosophical Essays on Freud*, R. Wollheim & J. Hopkins (eds), 289–305. Cambridge: Cambridge University Press.

Dawes, S. 1925. "Immigration and the Problem of the Alien Insane". *American Journal of Psychiatry* **81**: 449–70.

De Angelis, C., J. Drazen, F. Frizelle *et al.* 2004. "Clinical Trial Registration: A Statement from the International Committee of Medical Journal Editors". *Annals of Internal Medicine* **141**: 477–8.

DeLisi, L. E. & H. A. Nasrallah 1995. "Current Controversies in Schizophrenia Reaearch. I: Is Schizophrenia a Heterogeneous Disorder?". *Schizophrenia Research* **17**: 133.

De Sousa, R. 1984. "The Natural Shiftiness of Natural Kinds". *Canadian Journal of Philosophy* **14**: 561–80.

Descartes, R. [1641] 1968. *Meditations*. In *Discourse on Method and the Meditations*. Harmondsworth: Penguin.

Deutsch, A. 1944. "The First US Census of the Insane (1840) and its Use as Pro-slavery Propaganda". *Bulletin of the History of Medicine* **15**: 469–82.

Dimsdale, J., G. Klerman & J. Shershow 1979. "Conflict in Treatment Goals between Patients and Staff". *Social Psychiatry and Psychiatric Epidemiology* **14**: 1–4.

Drazen, J. & D. Zarin 2007. "Salvation by Registration". *New England Journal of Medicine* **356**(2): 184–5.
Duhem, P. 1954. *The Aim and Structure of Physical Theory*. Princeton, NJ: Princeton University Press. First published in French in 1914.
Dupré, J. 1981. "Natural Kinds and Biological Taxa". *The Philosophical Review* **90**: 66–90.
Dupré, J. 1993. *The Disorder of Things*. Cambridge, MA: Harvard University Press.
Dyson, W. & M. Mendelson 1968. "Recurrent Depressions and the Lithium Ion". *American Journal of Psychiatry* **125**: 544–8.
Ebersbach, A., M. Glaser & R. Heigl 2006. *Wiki – Web Collaboration*. Berlin: Springer.
Eisenberg, D. & G. Rozan 1960. "Mood Elevating Effects of Chlorphenoxamine HCl". *American Journal of Psychiatry* **117**: 155.
Ellis, B. 2001. *Scientific Essentialism*. Cambridge: Cambridge University Press.
Ellis, B. 2002. *The Philosophy of Nature*. Chesham: Acumen.
Emergency Medicine Journal Supplement 2006. "Life After Darkness – Cathy Wield". *Emergency Medicine Journal Supplement* (March): 2, http://emj.bmj.com/cgi/data/23/3/DC1/1.
Fernando, S. 2002. *Mental Health, Race and Culture*, 2nd edn. Basingstoke: Palgrave Macmillan.
Ferris, A. 1909. "Italian Immigration and Insanity". *American Journal of Insanity* **65**: 717–29.
Feyerabend, P. 1970. "Consolations for the Specialist". In *Criticism and the Growth of Knowledge*, I. Lakatos & A. Musgrove, 197–230. Cambridge: Cambridge University Press.
Fletcher, R. & J. Ungoed-Thomas 2005. "Food Labels of Confusion at Tesco". *Sunday Times* (27 February).
Flew, A. 1973. *Crime or Disease?* London: Macmillan.
Fodor, J. 1974. "Special Sciences (or The Disunity of Science as a Working Hypothesis)". *Synthese* **28**: 97–115.
Food Standards Agency 2004a. "Survey of Pizzas", Food Survey Information Sheet 58/04, www.food.gov.uk/science/surveillance/fsis2004branch/fsis5804.
Food Standards Agency 2004b. "Survey on basmati rice", Food Survey Information Sheet 47/04, www.food.gov.uk/science/surveillance/fsis2004branch/fsis4704basmati.
Food Standards Agency 2004c. "Survey on the Fat Content in Minced Meat", Food Survey Information Sheet 66/04, www.food.gov.uk/science/surveillance/fsis2004branch/fsis6604.
Foot, P. 2001. *Natural Goodness*. Oxford: Clarendon Press.
Foucault, M. 1970. *The Order of Things*. London: Tavistock.
Foucault, M. 1971. *Madness and Civilisation*. London: Tavistock. First published in French as *Histoire de la Folie* in 1961. First published in English in 1967.
Foucault, M. 1972. *The Archaeology of Knowledge*. London: Tavistock.
Foucault, M. 1976. *The Birth of the Clinic*. London: Tavistock.
Foucault, M. 2006. *History of Madness*. London: Routledge.
Freeman, W. & J. Watts 1950, *Psychosurgery in the Treatment of Mental Disorders and Intractable Pain*, 2nd edn. Oxford: Blackwell. First published 1942.
Freud, S. [1909] 1991. *Case Histories II*. Harmondsworth: Penguin.
Fuchs, S. 2001. *Against Essentialism*. Cambridge, MA: Harvard University Press.
Fulford, K. W. M. 1989. *Moral Theory and Medical Practice*. Cambridge: Cambridge University Press.
Fulford, K. W. M., T. Thornton & G. Graham 2006. *Oxford Textbook of Philosophy and Psychiatry*. Oxford: Oxford University Press.
Galison, P. 1997. *Image and Logic: A Material Culture of Microphysics*. Chicago, IL: University of Chicago Press.

Gendler, T. & J. Hawthorne 2005. "The Real Guide to Fake Barns: A Catalogue of Gifts for your Epistemic Enemies". *Philosophical Studies* **124**: 331–52.

Gilbody, S. & F. Song 2000. "Publication Bias and the Integrity of Psychiatry Research". *Psychological Medicine* **30**: 253–58.

Gilbody, S., A. House & T. Sheldon 2003. "Outcomes Measurement in Psychiatry: A Critical Review of Outcomes Measurement in Psychiatric Research and Practice", CRD Report 24. York: NHS Centre for Reviews and Dissemination, University of York.

Glasby, J. & P. Beresford 2006. "Who Knows Best? Evidence-based Practice and the Service User Contribution". *Critical Social Policy* **26**: 268–84.

Goldberg, T. E. & D. R. Weinberger 1995. "A Case Against Subtyping in Schizophrenia". *Schizophrenia Research* **17**: 147–52.

Goldman, A. 1976. "Discrimination and Perceptual Knowledge". *Journal of Philosophy* **73**: 771–91.

Goldman, A. 2006. *Simulating Minds*. Oxford: Oxford University Press.

Gordan, R. 1995. "Folk Psychology as Simulation". In *Folk Psychology*, M. Davies & T. Stone (eds), 60–73. Oxford: Blackwell. First published 1986.

Gould, S. J. 1981. *The Mismeasure of Man*. Harmondsworth: Penguin.

Grant, D. & E. Harari 2005. "Psychoanalysis, Science and the Seductive Theory of Karl Popper". *Australian and New Zealand Journal of Psychiatry* **39**: 446–52.

Greene, J. 2004. "Attention to 'Details': Etiquette and the Pharmaceutical Salesman in Postwar America". *Social Studies of Science* **34**: 271–92.

Grünbaum, A. 1984. *The Foundations of Psychoanalysis*. Berkeley, CA: University of California Press.

Gulliver, P., E. Peck & D. Towell 2002. "Balancing Professional and Team Boundaries in Mental Health Services: Pursuing the Holy Grail in Somerset". *Journal of Interprofessional Care* **16**: 359–70.

Hacking, I. 1986. "Making up People". In *Reconstructing Individualism*, T. Heller, M. Sosna & D. Wellberry (eds), 222–36. Stanford, CA: Stanford University Press.

Hacking, I. 1988. "The Sociology of Knowledge about Child Abuse". *Noûs* **22**: 53–63.

Hacking, I. 1992. "World-making by Kind-making: Child Abuse for Example". In *How Classification Works*, M. Douglas & D. Hull (eds), 180–238. Edinburgh: Edinburgh University Press.

Hacking, I. 1995a. *Rewriting the Soul*. Princeton, NJ: Princeton University Press.

Hacking, I. 1995b. "The Looping Effects of Human Kinds". In *Causal Cognition*, D. Sperber, D. Premack & A. Premack (eds), 351–94. Oxford: Clarendon Press.

Hacking, I. 1997. "Taking Bad Arguments Seriously: Ian Hacking on Psychopathology and Social Construction". *London Review of Books* (21 August): 14–16.

Hacking, I. 1998. *Mad Travelers*. Cambridge, MA: Harvard University Press.

Hacking, I. 1999. *The Social Construction of What?* Cambridge, MA: Harvard University Press.

Hamilton, B., E. Manias, P. Maude, T. Marjoribanks & K. Cook 2004. "Perspectives of a Nurse, a Social Worker and a Psychiatrist Regarding Patient Assessment in Acute Inpatient Psychiatry Settings: A Case Study Approach". *Journal of Psychiatric and Mental Health Nursing* **11**: 683–89.

Haraway, D. 1989. *Primate Visions: Gender, Race, and Nature in the World of Modern Science*. London: Routledge.

Haslam, N. 2002. "Kinds of Kinds: A Conceptual Taxonomy of Psychiatric Categories". *Philosophy, Psychiatry, & Psychology* **9**: 203–17.

Hayes, N. 1995. *Psychology in Perspective*. Basingstoke: Macmillan.

Heal, J. 2003. *Mind, Reason and Imagination*. Cambridge: Cambridge University Press.

Healy, D. 1990. *The Suspended Revolution*. London: Faber.

Healy, D. 1997. *The Antidepressant Era*. Cambridge, MA: Harvard University Press.

Healy, D. 2002. *The Creation of Psychopharmacology*. Cambridge, MA: Harvard University Press.

Healy, D. 2003. "In Debate with M. Thase: Is Academic Psychiatry for Sale?". *British Journal of Psychiatry* **182**: 388–90.

Healy, D. 2004. "Shaping the Intimate: Influences of the Experience of Everyday Nerves". *Social Studies of Science* **34**: 219–45.

Healy, D. & D. Cattell 2003. "Interface Between Authorship, Industry and Science in the Domain of Therapeutics". *British Journal of Psychiatry* **183**: 22–7.

Heil, J. & A. Mele (eds) 1993. *Mental Causation*. Oxford: Oxford University Press.

Hellewell, J. 2002. "Patients' Subjective Experiences of Antipsychotics". *CNS Drugs* **16**: 457–71.

Helmreich, S. 2005. "How Scientists Think; about 'Natives', for example. A Problem of Taxonomy among Biologists of Alien Species in Hawaii". *Journal of the Royal Anthropological Institute* **11**: 107–28.

Hiscock, J. & M. Pearson 1999. "Looking Inwards, Looking Outwards: Dismantling the 'Berlin Wall' Between Health and Social Services?" *Social Policy and Administration* **33**: 150–63.

Hoffman, M. 2000. *Empathy and Moral Development: Implications for Caring and Justice*. Cambridge: Cambridge University Press.

Hudson, J. & H. Pope 1990. "Affective Spectrum Disorder: Does Antidepressant Response Identify a Family of Disorders with a Common Pathophysiology?" *American Journal of Psychiatry* **147**: 552–64.

Humber, J. & R. Almeder (eds) 1997. *What is Disease?* Totowa, NJ: Humana.

Hurley, S. 2005. "The Shared Circuits Hypothesis: A Unified Functional Architecture for Control, Imitation and Simulation". In *Perspectives on Imitation: From Neuroscience to Social Science*, vol 1, S. Hurley & N. Chater (eds), 177–93. Cambridge, MA: MIT Press.

International Conference on Harmonisation of Technical Requirements for Registration of Pharmaceuticals for Human Use (ICH) 1996. *Guideline for Good Clinical Practice E6 (R1)*, www.ich.org/LOB/media/MEDIA482.pdf.

International Conference on Harmonisation of Technical Requirements for Registration of Pharmaceuticals for Human Use (ICH) Global Cooperation Group 2000. *Questions and Answers about ICH*, www.ich.org/LOB/media/MEDIA406.pdf.

International Committee of Medical Journal Editors (ICMJE) 2006. *Uniform Requirements for Manuscripts Submitted to Biomedical Journals: Writing and Editing for Biomedical Publication*, www.icmje.org/index.html#author.

Jardine, N., J. Secord & E. Spary (eds) 1996. *Cultures of Natural History*. Cambridge: Cambridge University Press.

Jarvis, E. 1852. "Insanity Among the Colored Population of the Free States". *American Journal of Insanity* **8**: 268–82.

Jaspers, K. [1913] 1974. "Causal and 'Meaningful' Connections Between Life History and Psychosis", J. Hoenig (trans.). In *Themes and Variations in European Psychiatry*, S. Hirsch & M. Shepherd (eds), 80–93. Bristol: Wright. Also available on the CD of readings that accompanies Fulford *et al.* (2006).

Jaspers, K. [1923] 1963. *General Psychopathology*, J. Hoenig & M. Hamilton (trans., German 7th edn). Manchester: Manchester University Press.

Kafka, J. & K. Gaarder 1964. "Some Effects of the Therapist's LSD Experience on his Therapeutic Work". *American Journal of Psychotherapy* **18**: 236–43.

Kandel, E. 1998. "A New Intellectual Framework for Psychiatry". *American Journal of Psychiatry* 155: 457–69.
Katz, R. 2004. "FDA: Evidentiary Standards for Drug Development and Approval". *NeuroRx* **1**: 307–16.
Kendler, K. 2001. "A Psychiatric Dialogue on the Mind–Body Problem". *American Journal of Psychiatry* **158**: 989–1000.
Kendler, K. 2005. "Toward a Philosophical Structure for Psychiatry". *American Journal of Psychiatry* **162**: 433–40.
Kim, J. 1993. *Supervenience and Mind*. Cambridge: Cambridge University Press.
Kirk, R. 2003. *Mind and Body*. Chesham: Acumen.
Kirsch, I., T. Moore, A. Scoboria & S. Nicholls 2002. "The Emperor's New Drugs: An Analysis of Antidepressant Medication Data Submitted to the US Food and Drug Administration". *Prevention and Treatment* **5**: article 23.
Klein, D. & M. Fink 1962. "Psychiatric Reaction Patterns to Imipramine". *American Journal of Psychiatry* **119**: 432–38.
Knowles, C. 2000. *Bedlam on the Streets*. London: Routledge.
Koertge, N. 2000. "Science, Values and the Value of Science. *Philosophy of Science* **67** (Proceedings): S45–S57.
Krafft-Ebing, von R. [1886] 1998. *Psychopathia Sexualis*. New York: Arcade.
Kripke, S. 1980. *Naming and Necessity*, rev. edn. Oxford: Blackwell.
Kuhn, T. 1970. *The Structure of Scientific Revolutions*. Chicago, IL: University of Chicago Press. First published 1962.
Ladd, P., M. Gulliver & S. Batterbury 2003. "Reassessing Minority Language Empowerment from a Deaf Perspective: The Other 32 Languages". *Deaf Worlds* **19**: 6–32.
Lagnado, M. 2003. "Increasing the Trust in Scientific Authorship". *British Journal of Psychiatry* **183**: 3–4.
Laing, R. D. 1965. *The Divided Self*. Harmondsworth: Penguin. First published 1959.
Laing, R. D. 1967. *The Politics of Experience and the Bird of Paradise*. Harmondsworth: Penguin.
Laing, R. D. & A. Esterson 1970. *Sanity, Madness and the Family*. Harmondsworth: Penguin. First published 1964.
Lakoff, A. 2005. *Pharmaceutical Reason: Knowledge and Value in Global Psychiatry*. Cambridge: Cambridge University Press.
Lenert, L., J. Ziegler, T. Lee, R. Sommi & R. Mahmoud 2000. "Differences in Health Values among Patients, Family Members and Providers for Outcomes in Schizophrenia". *Medical Care* **38**: 1011–21.
Lewis, R. 2004. "Should Cognitive Deficit be a Diagnostic Criterion for Schizophrenia?" *Journal of Psychiatry and Neuroscience* **29**: 102–13.
Lilienfeld, S. & L. Marino 1995. "Mental Disorder as a Roschian Concept: A Critique of Wakefield's 'Harmful Dysfunction' Analysis". *Journal of Abnormal Psychology* **104**: 411–20.
Longino, H. 1990. *Science as Social Knowledge: Values and Objectivity in Scientific Inquiry*. Princeton, NJ: Princeton University Press.
Loring, M. & B. Powell 1988. "Gender, Race, and DSM-III: A Study of the Objectivity of Psychiatric Diagnostic Behaviour". *Journal of Health and Social Behaviour* **29**: 1–22.
Luhrmann, T. 2000. *Of Two Minds: The Growing Disorder in American Psychiatry*. New York: Knopf.
Lukács, G. [1923] 1971. "Reification and the Consciousness of the Proletariat". In his *History and Class Consciousness*, R. Livingstone (trans.), 83–222. London: Merlin.
Lunbeck, E. 1994. *The Psychiatric Persuasion*. Princeton, NJ: Princeton University Press.

Macdonald, J. & J. Galvin 1956. "Experimental Psychotic States". *American Journal of Psychiatry* **112**: 970–76.
Mackay, L. 1993. *Conflicts in Care: Medicine and Nursing*. London: Chapman & Hall.
Malzberg, B. 1935. "Mental Disease among Foreign-born Whites, with Special Reference to Natives of Russia and Poland". *American Journal of Psychiatry* **92**: 627–40.
Malzberg, B. 1936. "Mental Disease among Native and Foreign-born Whites in New York State". *American Journal of Psychiatry* **93**: 127–37.
Marks, I. & R. Nesse 1994. "Fear and Fitness: An Evolutionary Analysis of Anxiety Disorders". *Ethology and Sociobiology* **15**, 247–61.
Marzillier, J. 2004. "The Myth of Evidence-based Psychotherapy". *The Psychologist* **17**: 392–5.
May, J. 1913. "Statistical Studies of the Insane". *American Journal of Insanity* **70**: 427–39.
McGinn, C. 1991. "Mental States, Natural Kinds and Psychophysical Laws". In his *The Problem of Consciousness*, 126–52. Oxford: Blackwell. First published 1978.
McGuire-Snieckus, R., R. McCabe & S. Priebe 2003. "Patient, Client or Service User? A Survey of Patient Preferences of Dress and Address of Six Mental Health Professions". *Psychiatric Bulletin* **27**: 305–8.
Mealey, L. 1995. "The Sociobiology of Sociopathy: An Integrated Evolutionary Model". *Behavioural and Brain Sciences* **18**, 523–41.
Megone, C. 1998. "Aristotle's Function Argument and the Concept of Mental Illness". *Philosophy, Psychiatry, & Psychology* **5**: 187–201.
Megone, C. 2000. "Mental Illness, Human Function and Values". *Philosophy, Psychiatry, & Psychology* **7**: 45–65.
Mill. J. S. [1843] 1973. *A System of Logic: Collected Works of John Stuart Mill, vol. VII*, J. Robson (ed.). Toronto, OT: University of Toronto Press.
Miller, L., D. Bergstrom, H. Cross. J. Herbert & J. Grube 1981. "Opinions and Use of the DSM System by Practicing Psychologists". *Professional Psychology* **12**: 385–90.
Miresco, M. & L. Kirmayer 2006. "The Persistence of Mind–Brain Dualism in Psychiatric Reasoning about Clinical Scenarios". *American Journal of Psychiatry* **163**: 913–18.
Molyneaux, J. 2001. "Interprofessional Teamworking: What Makes Teams Work Well?". *Journal of Interprofessional Care* **15**: 29–35.
Moos, R., A. Nichol & B. Moos 2002. "Global Assessment of Functioning Ratings and the Allocation and Outcomes of Mental Health Services". *Psychiatric Services* **53**: 730–37.
Murphy, D. 2006. *Psychiatry in the Scientific Image*. Cambridge, MA: MIT Press.
Nagel, E. 1961. *The Structure of Science*. London: Routledge & Kegan Paul.
Nagel, E. 1979. "Theory and Observation". In his *Teleology Revisited and Other Essays in the History and Philosophy of Science*, 29–48. New York: Columbia University Press. First published 1971.
National Committee for Mental Hygiene 1945. *Statistical Manual for the Use of Hospitals for Mental Diseases*, 10th edn. New York: National Committee for Mental Hygiene.
Nesse, R. 1987. "An Evolutionary Perspective on Panic Disorder and Agoraphobia". *Ethology and Sociobiology* **8**: 73S–83S.
Okun, R. 1970. "General Principles of Clinical Pharmacology and Psychopharmacology and Early Clinical Drug Evaluations". In *Principles of Psychopharmacology*, W. Clark & J. del Giudice (eds), 381–90. New York: Academic Press.
O'Malley, M. 1914. "Psychoses in the Colored Race". *American Journal of Insanity* **71**: 309–37.
Ortiz, D. 2001. "The Survivor's Perspective: Voices from the Center". In *The Mental Health Consequences of Torture*, E. Gerrity, T. Keane & F. Tuma (eds), 13–34. Dordrecht: Kluwer.

Parker, G., G. Gladstone & K. Chee 2001. "Depression in the Planet's Largest Ethnic Group: The Chinese". *American Journal of Psychiatry* **158**: 857–64.

Parker, M. 2005. "False Dichotomies: EBM, Clinical Freedom, and the Art of Medicine". *Medical Humanities* **31**: 23–30.

Parry, G. 2000. "Evidence Based Psychotherapy: Special Case or Special Pleading?". *Evidence-Based Mental Health* **3**: 35–7.

Pasamanick, B. 1962. "A Survey of Mental Disease in an Urban Population VII: An Approach to Total Prevalence by Race". *American Journal of Psychiatry* **119**: 299–305.

Peck, E. & I. Norman 1999. "Working Together in Adult Community Mental Health Services: Exploring Inter-professional Role Relations". *Journal of Mental Health* **8**: 231–42.

Perkins, R. 2001. "What Constitutes Success?". *British Journal of Psychiatry* **179**: 9–10.

Perlis, R., C. Perlis, Y. Wu, C. Hwang, M. Joseph & A. Nierenberg 2005. "Industry Sponsorship and Financial Conflict of Interest in the Reporting of Clinical Trials in Psychiatry". *American Journal of Psychiatry* **162**: 1957–60.

Pickstone, J. 2000. *Ways of Knowing*. Manchester: Manchester University Press.

Place, U. T. 1956. "Is Consciousness a Brain Process?". *British Journal of Psychology* **47**: 44–50.

Popper, K. 1959. *Logic of Scientific Discovery*. London: Hutchinson.

Popper, K. 1963. *Conjectures and Refutations*. London: Routledge & Kegan Paul.

Putnam, H. 1970. "Is Semantics Possible?". In his *Mind, Language and Reality*, 139–52. Cambridge: Cambridge University Press.

Putnam, H. 1975. "The Nature of Mental States". In his *Mind, Language and Reality: Philosophical Papers, vol. 2*, 429–40. Cambridge: Cambridge University Press. First published as "Psychological Predicates" in 1967.

Quine, W. V. O. 1960. *Word and Object*. Cambridge, MA: MIT Press.

Quine, W. V. O. 1961. "Two Dogmas of Empiricism". In his *From a Logical Point of View*, 20–46. New York: Harper & Row. First published 1951.

Radden, J. (ed.) 2004. *The Philosophy of Psychiatry: A Companion*. Oxford: Oxford University Press.

Ranney, M. 1850. "On Insane Foreigners". *American Journal of Insanity* 7: 53–63.

Rapley, M. 2004. *The Social Construction of Intellectual Disability*. Cambridge: Cambridge University Press.

Ravenscroft, I. 1998. "What is it Like to be Someone Else? Simulation and Empathy". *Ratio* **11**: 170–85.

Ray, I. 1849. "The Statistics of Insane Hospitals". *American Journal of Insanity* **6**: 23–52.

Regehr, C., G. Goldberg & J. Hughes 2002. "Exposure to Human Tragedy, Empathy and Trauma in Ambulance Paramedics". *American Journal of Orthopsychiatry* **72**: 505–13.

Reznek, L. 1987. *The Nature of Disease*. London: Routledge & Kegan Paul.

Reznek, L. 1991. *The Philosophical Defence of Psychiatry*. London: Routledge.

Richardson, R. 1984. "Biology and Ideology: The Interpenetration of Science and Values". *Philosophy of Science* **51**: 396–420.

Ripley, H. & S. Wolf 1947. "Mental Illness among Negro Troops Overseas". *American Journal of Psychiatry* **103**: 499–512.

Roberts, G. 2000. "Narrative and Severe Mental Illness: What Place do Stories have in an Evidence-based World?". *Advances in Psychiatric Treatment* **6**: 432–41.

Rogow, A. 1971. *The Psychiatrists*. London: Allen & Unwin.

Romme, M. & S. Escher 1993. *Accepting Voices*. London: Mind.

Rosanoff, A. 1915. "Some Neglected Phases of Immigration in Relation to Insanity". *American Journal of Insanity* **72**: 45–58.

Rosch, E. 1975. "Principles of Categorization". In *Cognition and Categorization*, E. Rosch & B. Lloyd (eds), 27–48. Hillsdale, NJ: Lawrence Erlbaum

Rose, H. 1987. "Hand, Brain and Heart: A Feminist Epistemology for the Natural Sciences". In *Sex and Scientific Inquiry*, S. Harding & J. O'Barr (eds), 265–82. Chicago, IL: University of Chicago Press. First published 1983.

Rosenhan, D. 1973. On Being Sane in Insane Places". *Science* **179**: 250–58.

Roth, A. & P. Fonagy 1996. *What Works for Whom?* New York: Guilford.

Ruse, M. 1981. "Are Homosexuals Sick?". In *Concepts of Health and Disease: Interdisciplinary Perspectives*, A. Caplan, H. Engelhardt & J. J. McCartney (eds), 693–723. Reading, MA: Addison-Wesley.

Sadler, J. 2005. *Values and Psychiatric Diagnosis*. Oxford: Oxford University Press.

Safer, D. 2002. "Design and Reporting Modifications in Industry-sponsored Comparative Psychopharmacology Trials". *Journal of Nervous and Mental Disease* **190**: 583–92.

Salmon, T. 1907. "The Relation of Immigration to the Prevalence of Insanity". *American Journal of Insanity* **64**: 53–71.

Saxena, S., I. Levav, P. Maulik & B. Saraceno 2003. "How International are the Editorial Boards of Leading Psychiatric Journals?". *Lancet* **361** (15 February): 609.

Schafer, A. 2004. "Biomedical Conflicts of Interest: A Defence of the Sequestration Thesis – Learning from the Cases of Nancy Olivieri and David Healy". *Journal of Medical Ethics* **30**: 8–24.

Schermerhorn, R. 1956. "Psychiatric Disorders Among Negroes: A Sociological Note". *American Journal of Psychiatry* **112**: 878–82.

Schiebinger, L. 2003. "Women's Health and Clinical Trials". *Journal of Clinical Investigation* **112**: 973–7.

Schiff, S. 2006. "Know it all – Can Wikipedia Conquer Expertise?" *New Yorker* (31 July).

Schoenwald S. & K. Hoagwood 2001. "Effectiveness, Transportability, and Dissemination of Interventions: What Matters When?". *Psychiatric Services* **52**: 1190–97.

Secord, A. 1996. "Artisan Botany". In *Cultures of Natural History*, N. Jardine, J. Secord & E. Spary (eds), 378–93. Cambridge: Cambridge University Press.

Seward, A. 2005. "Q & A: Intelligent Design". *Guardian* (30 September).

Shapin, S. & S. Schaffer 1985. *Leviathan and the Air-Pump*. Princeton, NJ: Princeton University Press.

Slater, L. 2004. *Opening Skinner's Box*. London: Bloomsbury.

Slater, L. 2005. "Reply to Spitzer and Colleagues". *Journal of Nervous and Mental Disease* **193**: 743–4.

Smart, J. J. C. 1959. "Sensations and Brain Processes". *Philosophical Review* **68**: 141–56.

Sorensen, R. 1998. "Self-strengthening Empathy". *Philosophy and Phenomenological Research* **58**: 75–98.

Speak, G. 1990. "An Odd Kind of Melancholy: Reflections in the Glass Delusion in Europe (1440–1680)". *History of Psychiatry* **1**: 191–206.

Spitzer, R., S. Lilienfeld & M. Miller 2005. "Rosenhan Revisited: The Scientific Credibility of Lauren Slater's Pseudopatient Diagnosis Study". *Journal of Nervous and Mental Disease* **193**: 734–9.

St Clair, H. 1951. "Psychiatric Interview Experiences with Negroes". *American Journal of Psychiatry* **108**: 113–19.

Stanley, N., B. Penhale, D. Riordan, R. Barbour & S. Holden 2003. "Working on the Interface: Identifying Professional Responses to Families with Mental Health and Child-care Needs". *Health and Social Care in the Community* **11**: 208–18.

Stanton, A. & M. Schwartz 1954. *The Mental Hospital*. New York: Basic Books.

Stevens, R. 1947. "Racial Aspects of Emotional Problems of Negro Soldiers". *American Journal of Psychiatry* **103**: 493–8.

Stone, E. & M. Priestley 1996. "Parasites, Pawns and Partners: Disability Research and the Role of Non-disabled Researchers". *British Journal of Sociology* **47**: 699–716.

Stueber, K. 2002. "The Psychological Basis of Historical Explanation". *History and Theory* **41**: 25–42.

Sumbre, G., Y. Gutfreund, G. Fiorito, T. Flash & B. Hochner 2001. "Control of Octopus Arm Extension by a Peripheral Motor Program". *Science* **293**: 1845–8.

Swift, H. 1913. "Insanity and Race". *American Journal of Insanity* **70**: 143–54.

Szasz, T. 1960. "The Myth of Mental Illness". *American Psychologist* **15**: 113–18.

Szasz, T. 1972. *The Myth of Mental Illness.* London: Paladin. First published 1961.

Telford, R. & A. Faulkner 2004. "Learning about Service User Involvement in Mental Health Research". *Journal of Mental Health* **13**: 549–59.

Thelmar, E. [1909] 1932. *The Maniac: A Realistic Study of Madness from the Maniac's Point of View*, 2nd edn. London: Watts.

Thomas, A. & S. Sillen 1972. *Racism and Psychiatry.* New York: Brunner/Mazel.

Thomas, P. & P. Bracken 2004. "Critical Psychiatry in Practice". *Advances in Psychiatric Treatment* **10**: 361–70.

Thornicroft, G., D. Rose, P. Huxley, G. Dale & T. Wykes 2002. "What are the Research Priorities of Mental Health Service Users?". *Journal of Mental Health* **11**: 1–3.

Townend, M. & T. Braithwaite 2002. "Mental Health Research – the Value of User Involvement". *Journal of Mental Health* **11**: 117–19.

Trivedi, P. & T. Wykes 2002. "From Passive Subjects to Equal Partners". *British Journal of Psychiatry* **181**: 468–72.

Tsuang, M. T. & S. V. Faraone 1995. "The Case for Heterogeneity in the Etiology of Schizophrenia". *Schizophrenia Research* **17**: 161–75.

Turner, M. 2003. "Psychiatry and the Human Sciences". *British Journal of Psychiatry* **182**: 472–4.

Tyrer, P. 2005. "Combating Editorial Racism in Psychiatric Publications". *British Journal of Psychiatry* **186**: 1–3.

Vaxevanis, A. & A. Vidalis 2005. "Cotard's Syndrome: A Three-case Report". *Hippokratia* **9**: 41–4.

Veterans Health Administration 1997. *Instituting Global Assessment of Function (GAF) Scores in Axis V for Mental Health Patients.* VHA Directive 97-059, 25 November 1997, www.avapl.org/gaf/gaf.html.

Von Wright, G. 1963. *The Varieties of Goodness.* London: Routledge & Kegan Paul.

Wagner, P. 1938. "A Comparative Study of Negro and White Admissions to the Psychiatric Pavilion of the Cincinnati General Hospital". *American Journal of Psychiatry* **95**: 167–83.

Wakefield, J. 1992a. "The Concept of Mental Disorder – On the Boundary Between Biological Facts and Social Value". *American Psychologist* **47**: 373–88.

Wakefield, J. 1992b. "Disorder as Harmful Dysfunction: A Conceptual Critique of DSM-III-R's Definition of Mental Disorder". *Psychological Review* **99**: 232–47.

Wakefield, J. 1999. "Evolutionary Versus Prototype Analyses of the Concept of Disorder". *Journal of Abnormal Psychology* **108**: 374–99.

Walmsley, J. 2001. "Normalisation, Emancipatory Research and Inclusive Research in Learning Disability". *Disability and Society* **16**: 187–205.

Widiger, T., A. Frances, H. Pincus, R. Ross, M. First & W. Davis (eds) 1994. *DSM-IV Sourcebook, vol. 1.* Washington, DC: American Psychiatric Association.

Widiger, T., A. Frances, H. Pincus, R. Ross, M. First & W. Davis 1996. *DSM-IV Sourcebook, vol. 2.* Washington, DC: American Psychiatric Association.

Widiger, T., A. Frances, H. Pincus, R. Ross, M. First & W. Davis 1997. *DSM-IV Sourcebook, vol. 3.* Washington, DC: American Psychiatric Association.

Wield, C. 2006. *Life After Darkness: A Doctor's Journey Through Depression.* Oxford: Radcliffe.

Wikipedia n.d. *Replies to Common Objections*, http://en.wikipedia.org/wiki/Wikipedia:Replies_to_common_objections.

Wilkerson, T. 1995. *Natural Kinds*. Aldershot: Avebury.

Wilkes, M., E. Milgrom & J. Hoffman 2002. "Towards more Empathic Medical Students: A Medical Student Hospitalization Experience". *Medical Education* **36**: 528–33.

Williams, D. & J. Garner 2002. "The Case against 'the Evidence': A Different Perspective on Evidence-based Medicine". *British Journal of Psychiatry* **180**: 8–12.

Wilson, D. & E. Lantz. 1957. "The Effect of Culture Change on the Negro Race in Virginia, as Indicated by a Study of State Hospital Admissions". *American Journal of Psychiatry* **114**: 25–32.

Wilson, J. & R. Thomas 2004. *Empathy in the Treatment of Trauma and PTSD.* New York: BrunnerRoutledge.

Winston, M. 1987. *Biology of the Honey Bee.* Cambridge, MA: Harvard University Press.

Wittgenstein, L. 1953. *Philosophical Investigations.* Oxford: Blackwell.

Wittgenstein, L. 1969. *On Certainty*. Oxford: Blackwell.

Wood, R. W. 1885. *Memorial of Edward Jarvis, MD.* Boston: T. R. Marvin.

Wright, L. 1973. "Functions". *Philosophical Review* **82**: 139–68.

Zachar, P. 2000. "Psychiatric Disorders are not Natural Kinds". *Philosophy, Psychiatry, & Psychology* 7: 167–82.

Zimmerman, M. 2005. "Pseudopatient or Pseudoscience: A Reviewer's Perspective". *Journal of Nervous and Mental Disease* **193**: 740–42.

Zimmerman, M., M. Posternak & I. Chelminski 2004. "Using a Self-report Depression Scale to Identify Remission in Depressed Outpatients". *American Journal of Psychiatry* **161**: 1911–13.

Index